The Many Dimensions of Dementia as Seen Through Family's Eyes. Subtitle: Family Reaches out to God for Guidance on Their Bumpy Ride.

Shirley KalpinOlson

Published by Shirley KalpinOlson, 2024.

The Many Dimensions of Dementia as Seen Through Family's Eyes

Subtitle: Family Reaches out to God fort Guidance on their Bumpy Ride.

By

Shirley KalpinOlson

THE MANY DIMENSIONS OF DEMENTIA As SEEN THROUGH FAMILY'S EYES'

Subtitle: Family reaches out to God for guidance on their bumpy ride.

This book is the work of the author of the factual account of family involvement in their loved ones dementia. Names, places and times are fictional. Written with permission.

The Index references obtained are public and may be copied as a guide to help others to understand the obstacles that many of the dementia-stricken have to face as they dwell with these horrible diseases.

Dedication

This story is dedicated to all those who helped and supported this family. Especially we give thanks and praise The Lord and Savior, Jesus who got them through their bumpy rollercoaster ride. We give God all the glory. Quotes from NJV and NKJV Bibles.

<u>Message from God:</u> "My child no matter what you face in life, don't let go of My hand. Every blessings assigned to you will come to you. It is I, God who holds your todays and tomorrows in the palm of my hands. So, don't give up, just call on Me if you lose your way I will get you back on track. Love God

Blessing to all who read this story. God inspired this story and Author is honored to be used as vessel to bring the words of this story to remind us how God will work in all our lives as we go through struggles and trials, if we just ask Him to ride along with us.

We give God all the Glory fo r the writings of this book.

Love in Christ, Author Shirley KalpinOlson

TABLE OF CONTENT

INDEXES

Prologue

After Sally finished grocery shopping, she was to meet her husband Joe who was waiting outside but when she got there Joe wasn't to be found. He must have gone to the car, she thought, so she ran with her cart to the car and searched all around, but no car and no Joe. Because of Joe's forgetfulness and getting lost easily, this really frightened Sally. She didn't know if the car was stolen with him in it or he had taken the car without a license and either way; this was certainly not good. She rushed back into the store to page Joe and search for him but still no Joe. This really worried Sally as she knew Joe was in his mid-stages of dementia and if he took the car, it was hard telling where he was, because he got lost when he drove and if he didn't take the car he was in terrible danger. She didn't know what to do she asked God, "where is he?" She was ready to call the police but a little voice inside her said, "call home first." She didn't think he'd be home; he usually doesn't know how to get home but she did call and sure enough he had gotten home safely over an hour after he apparently left her there. She didn't know if she should be angry or relieved, but she was very frustrated. She told her granddaughter, who was at their house, to ask for his keys and bring him along to get her from the grocery store where he left her stranded. This was the beginning of a long, bumpy, rollercoaster ride of their loved one's Dementia. God remained with them through the many years of this dementia nightmare.

Chapter1 Ambulance Ride

One wintry day in December of 2018, Sally was half dozing next to her 82-year-old husband, Joe, who was sleeping peacefully on his favorite recliner. Suddenly she was shocked awake by horrible garbling, and shuffling sound coming from her husband. She got up quickly, rushed over to him and found him face down on the floor shuffling trying to get up. Trying to get him to his feet, she realized his legs just would not work for him. His arms continued to flutter about, and he kept slurring and mumbling words she could not understand. He also could not understand her words. She knew she could not get him up by herself. Her first thought was. "Oh, my goodness, he's having a stroke."

Dialing 911 and knowing the danger of the situation she was barely able to talk as the operator responded, "This is 911, what can we help you with?"

Sally's voice talked but her mind was in a jumble, "My husband has fallen and I'm not able to get him up. He keeps mumbling and pushing around frantically, and it appears as if he is having a stroke. His legs are not working for him."

The operator said, "An ambulance is on the way, so stay on the phone and just try to keep him as sedate as possible. Does he is having any pain? Were you able to check for pulses and breathing problems?

"He has a very rapid irregular pulse and he's breathing with much difficulty. He is not able to respond to questions, he keeps ranting, raving and trying to get up and is very irrational. He doesn't understand me, and I can't understand him."

"Did he hit his head when he fell?"

"He bumped the back of his head on the seat of the recliner, but I don't think he was hurt. I don't see any bruises or bumps. He did fall a few weeks back and hit his head severely against a hard object and had several stitches in the back of his head. He has been complaining of pain in the area. His doctor checked it just a few days ago, and said it was healing well. He did have x-rays and scans at the time with no big problem showing."

"Help is on the way. Try to get him to lay down on the floor and keep him calm. Is he combative"

"He keeps pushing me away, but I'll keep him as quiet as possible."

"Okay, stay on phone until Ambulance comes. Has he had problems like this before?"

"He was diagnosed with mild case of Vascular Dementia when he fell before. He had a heart attack about 20 years ago and in 2003, he had repaired Aortic and abdominal aneurism and a history of many vascular problems. Okay, I see the Policeman is here now." She said as the police pushed open the door and came in.

"Good I'll let you go and good luck."

"Thank you for your help."

The police officer tried to get Joe in a chair to talk to him, but still unable to get answer, as Joe kept fighting anyone who tried to help him. When the Ambulance and medics came, it took three people to get him on a cart and strap him down so he could not hurt himself.

The Ambulance driver asked, "Is there a way to get to the ambulance without having to push him through the fresh snow piling up on your sidewalk?"

"Yes, go through the garage right out to the ambulance." Sally was certainly glad their neighbor had just plowed the driveway out, but she had a ping of guilt, why did I not get the sidewalk shoveled before this happened. "Oh, I can't do everything," she rationalized to herself.

As they pushed the cart out to the ambulance, Joe was still thrashing wildly, and mumbling and trying to get unbound. Sally tried to contain him, but she had to let the medics do their job, her tears, keep trying to come. The memories of the situation of her first husband's fatal ride in an ambulance keep intruding fresh in her mind. "Oh Lord, don't let me lose another husband," She prayed.

Through her clouded mind she heard the medic explain, "We're taking him to the Hospital Emergency Room, here in town." They proceeded to calm him down by starting IV's and a sedative. As he calmed down, Sally placed a kiss on his forehead as he weakly smiled with a crocked smile.

She said, "I love you and will meet you in the hospital in a little while. The medics and nurses will take good care of you."

Tears fell as she had to immediately turn away and let go, not knowing if she would see him alive again. All this seemed to bring back the tragic thoughts of her first husband's final exit.

Chapter 2 Sally's Anxiety

After the ambulance pulled away, Sally rushed into her house, tears un-relenting and stomach flipping in fear. She cried out to God, whom she knew would listen, "Why, God, why is this happening again" Please be with Joe and take care of him. I do not want to lose him, also"

Sally rushed into the bathroom splashed water on her already reddened and swelling eyes and face. Threw a brush through her short wavy graying hair, graying more by the minute. She grabbed her purse, winter coat and boots and rushed out to her old cold Buick, praying she could get through the harsh fresh winter snow falling fast and furious. "These terrible winters. I wish February would be gone!"

Sally's mind is still in turmoil. tears kept falling as her car trudged through the increased snow piles, as she headed toward the hospital not knowing what was to come. Her mind so jumbled all she could think of was "Why again, what am I doing so wrong that my loved ones keep getting ill and possibly dying on me.

Sally's past flashed before as if it were yesterday. Her first husband was diagnosed with cancer about this same time 20 years earlier, but it came back just as it happened yesterday. She had come home from church that fatal day and found him lying on the floor with no breath in him. She had known that he was deathly sick with two deadly cancers with no chance of having a long life, but that also was too soon. Wanting him to come to church with her that morning, but he said he felt too weak. She did not want to leave him, but knew she also needed consult from her church and God. She had felt so helpless then as she was feeling right now. "Please help me God to manage this situation and give me some peace and in all of this," she cried out to God once again.

She sensed this would be another life-changer if this were a stroke and along with his dementia, she had so many doubts. But I cannot think about that now, I have more important things to think about getting in to see my husband quickly. She was realizing that God got her through the first time, He would not give up on her now. That gave her some peace. Before she knew it, she was at the hospital emergency room entrance and plowing her car through the heavy snow into the first open spot she could get into. It was starting to get dark and with the continual heavy snowfall, she was not sure if she would get out, she may be here for a while. I just need to see my husband, right away.

As she jumped out of her car and rushed into the hospital ER and asked about Joe, the receptionist quickly led her in to see her husband. This cannot be good, she thought.

When Sally arrived at Joe's ER room, she noticed her husband fighting with the nurses as they were trying to put another IV into his vein. "He pulled the other one out, along with his other tubes and monitor during his agitation," his Nurse told Sally.

Sally ran up to him and put her hands on his cheeks and gave him a kiss on his forehead and said, "Your wife is here. Let the nurses get you IV back so they can get some medication to help you."

He turned to her and smiled his crooked smile and remained calm enough for the nurses to get the IV and all the tubes and monitors on him again and oxygen restarted. When the monitor was replaced, Sally noticed his heart was extremely fast and radical with many PVCS showing his blood pressure was incredibly low. Sally could see he was in serious trouble. The nurse gave him a sedative and something to calm his heart irregularity. Sally was happy for that because as a nurse she knew PVCs could cause the heart to stop and death could be imminent.

The doctor came in and said, I think you should call his children to come in as soon as they can. Your husband's condition is serious. He may not even make it through the night. We are concerned about his blood pressure and his heart rate. And he may have another stroke. His kidneys are showing signs of shutting down, from what is going on with his body. We will let you know more when we get the results back. We will talk to you, hopefully your children can get here soon so they will also hear. Why don't you have a cup of coffee and call his children right away? I can see you are genuinely concerned. He will be ok now as he settles down. The nurses and I will keep a close eye on him. You can come back whenever you feel. We will be done and have results soon."

"Thank you. Sally said to the doctor, it'll be good to relax, knowing he is being cared for."

"I'm going to let your children know you are here, and I will see you, later, Joe and take it easy on the nurses and behave yourself, OK? Love you." She said to her husband.

Sally then went into the emergency waiting room to call his children. She was anxious to talk to them, and let them know how serious this was and hopefully they would come in as soon as they could. She called the oldest daughter, June, as she knew she would be home from work and said, "I hate to call you with sad news, but your dad was brought to the city hospital ER by ambulance. He is very seriously sick, and the doctor suggested all his children come here as soon as possible. The doctor is overly concerned and feels he may have another stroke or even his heart may stop. His BP is incredibly low, and he also has other problems, as his kidneys are showing signs of shutting down. He has been given heart medication and sedatives to prevent stroke or even more heart damage. He is waiting for the results to come in and we will know more when you get here. Will you let the rest know and come as soon as you can? Right now, he is very restless. And every time he is restless, his Blood pressure goes down and his heart is unstable. We are really concerned. Thank you. Hopefully we will see you soon."

June was genuinely concerned as she said. "Ann, (second daughter) is here so we will be there in about half an hour."

"Your dad will appreciate that. I will be waiting in the ER waiting room. I am going to check on him now and will let you know more about his situation when you get here. Love you."

Chapter 3 Family Alerted

A half-hour later, the daughters June and Ann rushed into the ER waiting room where Sally was waiting.

They told Sally, "Our brother will be coming in later. How is dad doing? Can we see him?"

Sally knew they would be concerned and anxious to see their dad, so Sally had planned with his nurse to be able to see him when they came in. She told them, "Check at the nurse's station before you go in, he was given medication to help him rest. He has been very anxious and pulling at his tubes. He may be sleeping, and he needs his rest."

The girls checked at the desk and got their permission. When they entered their dad's room and walked over to him, he had just woken up from his rest. He looked at them as if he didn't recognize them and was unable to respond to them. When they took his hand and told him who they were, he still had a tough time recognizing they were his daughters. Tears flowed, to see their dad this way.

Sally could see the reaction. She went over to them and put her arm around them in support, saying, "He just awoke from a good sleep and sometimes medication causes this reaction. He will know you later when he's more awake."

The doctor also came in, and noticing the situation, said. "Yes. Right now, he is in a state of not sure where he is or what is going on. I have more answers about your dad's condition so let us let him wake up more while we go into my office so we can talk. While the nurses check him."

The family fearfully walked into Dr's office with Sally, as Joe's son, Ted, was led into the room.

The ER doctor said. "I am not going to mince words with you. Your dad is seriously ill. With his history of small strokes, he also has an unbelievably bad case of right lobe pneumonia, with sepsis, which is an infection of his blood. His body is also showing signs of shutting down. We are not sure the cause of the sepsis, but we are starting large doses of antibiotics which cover most bacterial sepsis infections and combining his antibiotics regime with copious amounts of fluids to maintain his blood pressure, we feel this is the only thing we can do now and see if the body functioning will retain to sustain life. The truth is he has an extremely poor prognosis. Also, with his history of heart attack, aortic aneurysm, and vascular disease complications, it is causing small strokes which can damage areas in the brain which may increase his dementia. If these small strokes increase, he may have a major stroke. He has been given medication to prevent the strokes for now. How long has he had this dementia?"

Sally was perplexed as she said, "His regular doctor diagnosed dementia, toward the end of September, about three months ago, after he had a fall and cut his head open, stitches needed. Since then, I noticed an increase in his symptoms. Do you think his extreme, rational, combative behavior and outbursts is from his dementia?"

"Yes," the doctor said, "the sepsis and pneumonia will decrease the oxygen to the brain which also increases dementia."

The family groaned, as they realized the seriousness of their dad's condition. They have many more questions. But the family said, "Thank you, doctor, for explaining all this to us. We had no idea what was in store. His Alzheimer's will gradually cause more confused, Is that right?"

"Yes, He will gradually increase to stranger and uncontrolled dementia. Remember this is not Alzheimer's which is one of the types or systems of dementia. There are many types of dementia. Your dad's type is

Vascular dementia, caused by his decrease of blood flow through the veins.

"Won't the extremely fluid pushing so fast be hard on his heart?" one of the daughters asked seeing the IV dripping fast.

"Yes, but we needed to load him with copious amounts of fluids as his kidneys were starting to shut down and blood pressure dropping dangerously low. He needs quiet time now and if he becomes combative, irrational, or restless as he tends to do, we will need to give him a sedative through his IV."

"Won't this medication drop his blood pressure and cause more problems? his son asked soberly.

"It may, but if he becomes irritated it would affect his heart. It is the lesser of the evils." The doctor said sadly, placing his hand on his shoulder in comfort.

When the family walked back onto the ER room, Sally, in all her nursing career, never was so frightened as to what was happening to her husband. She knew this was a profoundly serious situation. She watched the monitors closely, and noticed the increasing PVC'S which she was fearful of his heart giving up and his blood pressure of 50/30 she knew could be unsustainable. She knew everything was putting pressure on his heart. "Please God don't take another husband from me" Sally cried softly out to God.

The doctor and nurse came in again, as the doctor said. "We are going to transfer your dad and husband to ICU on 2nd floor. There is nothing more we can do for him, here. The nurses will be watching one on one, there. Why don't you all go to have coffee and when we get him settled into ICU, we will let you know

Chapter 4 Critical Diagnosis with Miracle

A half hour later the nurse notified the family their dad was in ICU, the doctor said, "Joe is in an extremely critical state, but his body needs rest now. He is in a semi-conscious state. We had to give more medication to calm him for now. You can all go in for just a brief time to let him know you are here, but do not stay too long. He is in such a critical state, rest for his body is especially important. His chance of getting through the night is only about 50/50%.

You may wait in the waiting room, if you want, but we only allow 1 person at a time in his room. He tends to become irrated with any stimuli. And rest is really what he needs now more than anything. It would be a better idea if you all went home to get rest. You are close enough we can notify you immediately if something should happen."

The siblings tearfully all said their goodbyes to their almost unconscious dad. and quietly walked out of the room tears flowing.

The family met in the ICU waiting room for a brief time. All had questions and searched for answers. Sally tried to comfort them with as many answers she had but she was so fearful she did not want to let on. They said a prayer together and Sally offered her house to stay in to be closer to their dad. They said they would be ok and just asked her to call them right away if anything happened.

After the family left, Sally went back to her husband's room to say a little prayer to him and say good night. She gave her husband a kiss on his cheek. He tried to move his hand toward her, but it fell limp on the bed. Tears flowed from Sally's check, as she ran from the room and gave the nurses her phone number so they could call her right away, if they needed her for anything

That night Sally was very apprehensive about her husband's critical condition. She laid wide awake, thinking and worrying. unable to sleep. As she looked at the clock it read 2AM, she suddenly heard a voice saying, "Pray for a miracle for your husband, to get through the night The Lord is a healing God."

Sally got down on her knees beside the bed, clasped her hands in prayer and prayed aloud, "Please God, my husband needs a miracle to get through the night, instead of a 50/50 chance to live, he needs a 100% healing. I cannot lose another husband. I need him in my life. I totally put him in your hands and reveal a sigh that you are healing his body. I trust you are a healing God. Thank you In Jesus name. Amen

After that prayer. She knew in her heart Jim would be better the next day. Confident in God, she was able to fall asleep with her phone by her side just in case the staff needed her.

That night Sally's dreams were filled with sweet dreams of her husband sitting up and joking with the nurses. He then asked them. "Could you get my britches, I need to get out of here."

After a good hard sleep full of wonderful dreams. Sally suddenly woke, startled. The clock read 8am and no phone call. She prayed, "I hope I did not miss a call. Then a little voice said, "do not be troubled, I gave you a sign in your dream." She knew God had worked a miracle in her husband. She quickly called the hospital and asked, "How is my husband doing this morning? Is he eating breakfast?

"As a matter of fact, he is, how did you know that he was better?"

"God told me in a dream. I will be coming to see him in a brief time. Thank you for reinforcing what God told me."

Sally happily called the family that their dad had miraculously made it through the night and was doing well. I am on my way there. I will let You know more when I get there."

Sally quickly dressed, brushed her hair, splashed water on her face and put on make-up, as she was praising the Lord.

She jumped in her used Buick. Lots of snow had filled the driveway, but Sally was able to plow through

with her heavy car. She was glad the roads were clear and not slippery. She got to the hospital without a problem. She knew God was traveling with her as she parked near the ICU entrance.

When she walked into the ICU room she gasped in glee. Joe was sitting up, in his bed. Tubes in all orifices, except his mouth, and his first words from there were, "Where are my britches? Il need to get out of here."

She laughed as she ran to him, kissed him on his cheek and said, "I knew you would make it through the night. God gave me a sign in my dream."

Joe smiled, through his still slightly crooked smile, and said, "Hallelujah and praise the Lord. But please find my britches."

Joe's daughters arrived about that time and could not believe their eyes at his tremendous turn-around. "How did he make such a quick recovery. I do not understand. I cannot believe he has gotten better so fast. It is a miracle." The daughters said.

The nurses and the doctor came in just at that minute and said, "Yes, we believe that Joe had a miracle. He changed around 2:00 AM during the night. His blood pressure had almost bottomed out earlier, but it completely changed to normal, almost immediately, after 2:00 am. He then asked for the britches he wanted to get out of there. We could not believe the fast change and the miracle."

Sally beamed with love as she said, "I know why. God gave us this miracle. Last night, at 2am, I was unable to sleep. I knew I needed to pray for a miracle. I was urged to get down on my knees to pray to our wonderful healing God. God heard these prayers. Then he gave me a wonderful dream that Joe would be sitting up joking with the nurses and asking them. 'Could you get my britches. I want to get out of here.' Those were the exact words he said to me when I came into his room this morning. I really do believe in the power of prayers." Sally stated.

"After hearing what you just told us, we also believe in the power of prayer," the Dr and nurses said in unison. All stood stunned that it was the same time as the prayers. And the same words from Joe. "God is so good" everyone said as they stood around Joe's bed and prayed in Thanksgiving for this great miracle.

As they were all rejoicing about the miracle. Joe spoke up "Okay, now, how about getting my britches."

Chapter 5 Joe's Life Change

"We will get your britches, but we are going to transfer you to another room on this floor after we take all your unnecessary tubes out. We will continue to keep you on a heart monitor, and you will be near the nurse's station. Your IV will remain in your vein to continue your antibiotics for a few more days, to help clear up your Pneumonia and sepsis, which is improving very well. Yes. God is giving you a healing. We just need to monitor you a little longer. If all goes well, you may be able get your britches on and go home in a few more days."

"Wow, which sounds great, right Joe." But quietly she said to the nurse, "I don't know if I will be able to manage him if he becomes agitated."

"We have already planned a patient care conference for 1pm tomorrow. And if you can get most of his siblings here to listen to the doctor and care- givers to make plans for his care while at home. They will be able to ask questions and understand his illness. They should be part of his care, also.

"That's great." said one of the daughters. "I'll get the rest of our family here at 1pm tomorrow."

"Yes, if you will that will certainly help out." Sally said.

"The family should all be part of their dad's care, whenever they can, especially with his increasing dementia." The nurse said.

The daughters left then, promising to be back the next day at 1pm, with their brother.

Sally stayed for a while with her hubby. Then as it was getting dark outside, and he was starting to fall asleep, she gave him a kiss on his lips, and told him. "I am going to leave for the night." Sally just realized she hadn't eaten since yesterday. "I promise I'll be back tomorrow morning."

"Okay." Joe weakly said as his eyes closed.

Sally went out to the desk and told his nurse I am going to leave. I am exhausted and haven't eaten since yesterday and will be back in the morning. He is sleeping now so keep a close eye on him. Thanks."

"Yes. We will keep a close eye on him from the desk and will take diligent care of him, so do not worry and get some well-deserved rest and food. We do not want you to get sick."

Sally left and got something to eat and went home, prayed a prayer of thanksgiving for her hubby's miracle and asked God to continue to heal her husband and give her strength and help to keep going herself. After praying she fell sound asleep through the whole night, knowing God was in control. The next morning, Sally called the hospital to check how her husband's night had gone.

The nurse told Sally, "He had a very restless night, so we placed him even closer to the nurses' station. He is sitting up in his chair now and waiting for PT to take him for a walk down the hall. He keeps looking for you and still asking for his britches. If you could bring them in with you, we could use them to pacify him, when you are not here. You can come in later this morning; we will keep him busy with PT and OT so hopefully he won't try to wander off. We plan his care plan for this afternoon. Will his family be here?"

"Yes. I talked to them this morning and they all plan to be here at 1:00. I will come in about 11:00. Please tell him I will be coming in later and I will not forget his britches. Thank you. I'll see you then."

"Ok, we plan to have all the people here to talk to him about his home cares. Before the family comes, we will explain that the children need to have a good relationship with all the others who will work with them so you will be able to go home soon. Hopefully he'll have an idea of the goings on, so he won't be alarmed by all the people showing up.

"Thanks for the loving care. See you soon,

Chapter 6 Family Care Conference

Sally busied herself with doing all the things she was not able to do earlier. She washed Joe's britches and packed clean socks and underwear to bring with her to the hospital. After a quick lunch, Sally backed out of her garage and noticed that the snow had piled up at the end of the driveway, so she had to shovel to get out of the driveway before heading back to the hospital.

Sally finally got to Joes room around 11 am. The nurse was putting him back in bed and said I do not know how he keeps sneaking out of his room, even after all his activities this morning. You think he would be worn out? We found him wandering down the hall ready to get on the elevator when we were able to find him. He kept saying, "I'm looking for my wife she's supposed to bring my britches."

"Joe, why do you keep wondering about? I told you I'd be here and bring your britches."

"I just needed my britches." he said, as his head hung down.

"Okay, we got your britches. Why don't you rest for a little after we get you all dressed up with clean britches and clothes before your family and all your visitors come in."

"Why are so many coming here?"

"You remember we are having a care conference where many people are coming to talk with you to tell you what their plans for you when you get out of the hospital."

"Can't I just go home with my wife."

"That's what we are having this meeting about, to see if you're able to go home." His nurse explained.

"I'm doing good I'll behave myself at home with my wife, if I have my britches and clothes to wear. " Joe said innocently.

Sally grinned and said, "Why don't you lie down for a little while before your children get here and you will be all ready for all your visitors to come in. We will have more answers then, about your coming home."

"OK. I will rest while you are here. I have already had my lunch. Did you eat?"

"Yes, I ate before I left, so I'll sit right next to you and rest until your family comes."

Around 1pm, Joes children walked in. Joe had taken a short nap, so he was more alert and happy to see them.

The nurse came in shortly and got Joe up and they all walked down the hall to the conference room. When the Nursing supervisor, Joe's doctor, his Physical and Occupational Therapists, the hospital Pharmacists, Social Service personnel and others came into the conference room, all very friendly to Joe. It looked like Joe was enjoying the friendliness and kindness of all. He felt like a king.

Then he asked, not remembering, "Why are you all here?"

The gal from Social Service said, "we're here to try and find the perfect place for you when you get out of the hospital, where you may need more help."

Then talking to Sally, she said. "We have checked places where we can send Joe to get more rehab before he can go home. Most are a long way from here toward the cities. The ones close by are all filled or do not accept memory care people."

"We're concerned about our dad, so what are we supposed to do or how to get him care?" June, the oldest daughter asked.

The gal from social service said, "Yes, we are also worried about where we can find a place to take him. Most if the places we have found even close by runs close to $3000-$5000. a month with little basic cares."

Sally said, "there's no way I could pay that, even using both of our total incomes."

"This is terrible. My dad has worked all his life and has spent 4 years in the Marines serving this country and now when he needs help, there is none for him. You see illegals break into this country and are put up in expensive hotels at our expense. Does not seem quite right," Ted said angrily

"I understand your anger and that certainly seems right. We have produced a plan which could work if we can get cooperation from his family to help Sally at times."

"We all have jobs, but we will help when we can. So, what is the plan?"

"We can send him to his own home with personnel such as nurses', OT, and others to work with him and Sally at the home at least three or four times every week they would coordinate their times to spend at least 1 hour, 1 or 2 times a day, every day. Then we could have meals on wheels come 3x's per week in between. The only times not covered would be weekends, which could be the hardest for Sally. We were hoping his children could pick up the pace by taking him for an hour or so a day or when she needs to get groceries etc. Maybe taking him for a night or part of a night so she can get rest."

"As your dad becomes more cognitive deficient, he may need protective measures in the home so he will not wander and fall down the stairs or wonder outside while Sally's sleeping. As his dementia increases, he will have more falls and will need people to help Sally get him up. Just be there to help as you all can." Joe's doctor said

"We do have a lot of good helpers that are very good people that come in to help him and he might even like that and especially because he'll be in his own home, he will feel more comfortable." Joe's nurse said.

Ted, Joe's son said, "Since we all have jobs, we could take turns helping during a weekend when we can. I am personally fearful of taking him to our house as he may become more frightened, confused, and wander off."

"Maybe if you can just come over to our home and just spend time and visit with him when you can. I can get the things I need to do while you are visiting. He would love that. He is always asking for you to see him."

"Or maybe just take him out for a meal to a restaurant or place he's familiar with and visit all together as a family." His nurse mentioned.

"In the middle of September and 2 weeks later, I am scheduled for both eye surgeries. I will need someone to stay with him overnight on both nights. I cannot take care of him when I get back. That is what they are telling me. I will be here at night, so if you leave in morning, I will be able to take care of after a nights' rest."

June, oldest daughter said, "I could do the first surgery and stay with dad. But I may be going back to work after that, so maybe someone else could come for the second surgery."

"Well, thanks for your sacrifices to help, your dad will love that because he will feel comfortable with you girls. Any help he can get from his family he will love." Sally says with a slight tear in her eyes.

Ted had questions for the pharmacy on his medicines if he would have become agitated when we take him. "What we going to do?" His son asked.

"We will give him a pill that he can take orally if he does need it, but we do not want to encourage it too often," The pharmacist stated.

"Maybe divert his attention to something he is familiar with. You live in the country, and he is a country boy he will catch on to seeing a horse or something. His biggest problem will be if he is left alone for any length of time." His doctor said

"I will have all his pills he may need while with you ready for him and labeled when he is supposed to have them and a separate pill box,

With a couple of relaxing pills, he may need for emergency. "Sally said.

"What do you think about all if these plans?" the doctor asked the family.

"I think. Joe, you will love all these people coming to see and visit with you in your own home, right?" Sally asked Joe.

"Right, I love when people come to visit me."

When the staff was ready to leave, the family all thanked them by saying. "We appreciate all the things you have told us and what you are doing to help our dad. We feel much more prepared for his future."

Sally thanked them all saying, "We know we will be okay as we travel this rollercoaster ride with our loved one, knowing that God will be traveling alongside us. He was there for Joe's healing. We know He will be with us now. All we need is to pray and believe and He will ride along with us."

Sally felt Joes' children understood the situation much better and she knew they would be fine as God was with them.

The family went back to Joes room after all the personnel left. Sally asked Joe, "What did you think of all your visitors and what they told us?"

"Who were all those people? Why were they there? I could not understand a word they were saying."

Sally and the family groaned. They all knew this rollercoaster ride would be a challenge. But Sally also knew God would be traveling with them. Later, while their dad was having his physical therapy and his dinner, the family and Sally went to the cafeteria to have dinner. When they returned to his room, they visited for a brief time with their dad and then said their goodbyes and left for the night.

Chapter 7 Sleep over

Sally stayed with Joe until the nurse came in to get him settled for the night. The nurse said. "We will give him a sedative. He has had a long day so he will rest better tonight, and we will be close by to watch him because we are right across the desk. So, you might as well go home and get some rest. And don't worry about your husband. Sally gave Joe a kiss and told him she would come back in the morning.

Sally headed to her car as darkness surrounded her. Snow was coming down so hard that she was hardly able to see her car. It was getting very, very cold as she rushed into the car and tried to start the car and it would not start. It just groined. She did not know what to do. The battery was completely dead on her old Buick. She ran into the hospital to ask the nurse, at the nurse's station, if there was somebody that could help her get her car started or have a jumper as her battery was dead. One of the securities came out and brought a portable Battery charger but would not even start to charge. No juice in battery.

It was 10pm. Very dark and extremely late. Sally knew she would not get anyone to help this late.

Sally went back into the hospital and told the nurse at the nurse's station her predicament.

The nurses said, "Why don't you sleep in your husband's room, and we will bring in a reclining chair. You could sleep in there for the night, and you can get someone to help you in the morning."

Sally was thankful for their help. Since Joe was resting quietly, she went to the nurses' lounge until they could get a chair for her.

She prayed," Lord, thank you for helping. I know you are here to get help with my Ole car in the morning. This car problem is now a problem I need help with, but I know you are a great helper in all trouble. Thank you for this help to come. This rollercoaster is starting and going faster but I know you are here to ride with us. Thank you in Jesus' name Amen

The staff brought a reclining chair into Joe's room shortly after and the nurse came and told Sally her bed was waiting for Sally to sleep beside her husband.

Sally thanked the nurse and crawled into the reclining comfortable chair without waking her sleeping husband. She was sound asleep before she knew it. When she awoke, she noticed her husband gazing at her with a smile on his face. She reached over to him and gave him a big hug.

"What are you doing here? I thought you were going home, but I am glad you are here."

"I was on my way home. But my car would not start. I have a dead battery. The security guard tried to charge it, but that did not help. I am going to call Carl, my son, to see if he could come over and give me a jump the Buick, from his car. And he can drive it home. We will have to pick up another battery. I do not want to take a chance on driving. I will find a way here tomorrow. But may have to stay overnight again tomorrow night."

"That will sure be all right with me," Joe said. "Happy to have you here. Now I will not have to go around looking for you."

The nurse came in about that time and said, "yes, that is right, he had an incredibly good night. Since you were here by his side, we did not hear a peep from him. You can stay any night you want. It helps him."

"I thought he had a good night, because I would have heard if he would have gotten out of bed, because normally I am a light sleeper, but last night I slept like a lamb and I did not wake up until he was staring at me. Wondering who I was, I think."

"Oh, I knew who you were," Joe said. "You are my wife. I could not forget you."

The nurse brought in Joe's tray with enough food on it for both. After they ate Sally dialed her son. When a groggy Carl answered, Sally said, "I am sorry to be calling so early. This is your mom; I am at the hospital here with Joe. Was not able to get my car started, last night, battery went dead, so I slept overnight here. Could you come with cables and give my car a boost as soon as you are able so I can get home? I would really appreciate it."

"OK, we will be there. If may take a while? We need to get dressed and get on the road. The roads may be slippery, it is rough out there, but do not worry, we will be there. See you in an hour or so."

"Thank you so much. I will wait here for now and be downstairs about an hour, just when you come, so I can show you where the car is parked snowed in."

Sally waited with Joe and took him for a walk. She then said goodbye to him with a kiss and said, "I am not sure when I will be back. Will need time to get battery etc. and car checked. You be good and do not give the nurses a tough time."

"I'll try."

The nurse came in and said to Joe, smiling, "You will have to behave, we are watching you. Besides if you try to get up a little buzzer goes off."

"Am I that special and important?"

"You sure are." The two said in unison, as Sally kissed his cheek and rushed out.

When she arrived down to where her car was her son and wife were already there placing cables on the car. The area had been plowed so they were able to spot the car.

Carl said "It is starting to take a charge so why don't you gals wait inside where it warm. I will wait here in the car and get you when I get it started."

"Sounds like a good plan, but make sure you stay warm in our car," his wife said shivering.

When Carl came in to where the gals were, he said, "Well, got it started, finally, but we are going to let it run and warm up for a while. It took a long time to get that battery built up. What did you do, Mom to get that battery so low?"

"Who, me? I am just a mom. I do not have any idea what a car does or does not do, but I really appreciate your knowledge. Thank you so much for the help."

"I will drive your car home when the car gets warmed up. I am going to stop and pick up a new battery and have it put in while there in case it stops again. My wife can take you home and get some rest. Looks like you are exhausted. I am sure all this is wearing on you."

"Yes, I am getting worn out, but if you pick up a battery it would be great. With a new battery, I should be able to start it in the morning. "

"I should hope it starts unless there is more wrong with it. I will see you both later." Carl said as he kissed both his mom and wife, on their cheeks.

"Thanks, I needed that," Sally said as they walked back out to the cars. Sally and her daughter-in-law jumped in their car and the two headed for her house, while Carl drove her old Buick.

It was going to be good to get home. She did not realize how exhausting everything was getting. When home, Sally told her daughter-in law, Sue what their plans for Joe, "The hospital personnel tried to find a rehab place for him when he gets out of the hospital, but everything close by were full and most places refused to take memory care patients."

"So, what are they going to do?" Sue asked"

"He will be coming home here, with home care. It means they will send nurses every 2-3 days for an hour at a time combining on other days with OT and PT. The only days I am concerned about is weekends. But his family were encouraged to take him for short times while on the weekends They said they will do what they can when they can. I think they may be afraid of their dads increase and changes of his dementia. He has gotten worse since his hospitalization." Sally said with sadness.

"Why don't you take a refreshing shower and crawl into your bed. I will just read my book and wait for Carl. I will give you a call tomorrow to see if you need a ride anywhere." car.

"Thanks," Sally showered and crawled into her bed. She prayed for Gods help on her car situation, and thanked God that her husband would be taken care of. It sounded like they would be watching him close. Sally prayed and thanked God for all the help, but she was still concerned about her car. That night Sally had a dream God told her not to worry He would send an angel to help her.

Next morning, Sally got up, and went out to the garage. Sure thing, the old Car would not start, so she stuck the battery charger on, but it would hardly move. Sally said a little prayer and called the hospital and said," I will not be able to come in this morning, am still having car problems, will be there this afternoon for Joe's second care conference at 2. How is Joe doing?"

"Joe is quieter today. He is worried about you. I will tell him you called and will here at 2 this afternoon. He has his britches and shoes on, so he is content for now," his nurse said laughing.

"Good. That will have to be his protocol when he comes home." It felt good for Sally to laugh.

Chapter 8 Car problem; Angel to The Rescue

After talking with the nurse Sally called Ted and thought, he works on cars he can do something with it. He may still have my old car he fixed before. Wouldn't it be wonderful if they would trade this one for my old one? I would not mind having my white car back. It might be a pipe dream. Sally was talking to God in her mind.

Sally called Ted and prayed, Lord, please help Ted can do something to help me. I just do not know if I can manage any more problems. I'm just so worn out. Then suddenly a little voice said to her, "That is OK. I told you in a dream that I am sending an Angel your way to help you."

When Ted answered Sally told him of the car problems and said, "even with a new battery it still would not start this morning the new battery is now dead. Do you know what could be causing this problem? I am supposed to be at the hospital at 2 for another care conference. I can get a bus there for now but will need wheels to get back and forth."

Ted said, "I will be right over and have my friend come and we can haul the car back here if we still cannot get the car to go. I will check with June if she would like the Buick and get your other car back. She does not like small cars. She may want to make a swap."

"You would do that for me? That would be a miracle."

Ted and his friend showed up before Sally had to call for a bus ride and said, "June and I talked, and she said she would like to swap cars. She likes Buicks, and you can have your Nissan back. You will have to get together sometime and exchange titles. How does that sound?"

"Thank you so much. You must be an angel." Sally was thrilled because she always liked her old car.

"Me an angel. I hardly think so. Why would you say that? Ted said laughing

"God told me in a dream, He was sending me an angel to help me. And you are my angel." She gave her stepson a hug

"Okay, would this angel like to give you a ride to the hospital, so you don't have to get a bus, before we haul your car away."

"That would be so nice of my angel. I will get a ride home on my own or Joe does not mind if I sleep in his room. Like I did two nights ago."

On the way to the hospital, Ted said, "We can bring your other car here tomorrow. Then you will have wheels again. When will dad be coming home?"

"We will know more today They are having a conference to go over plans. I will make a copy of all the plans and give you one for all. If one of your sisters would like to come with me when he comes home, that would be an immense help."

"I'll tell them, and you can let us know when he is able to get out."

"Wow, I will get my old car back, I cannot believe it. Thanks, do much for all your help." Sally said as she got out of Ted's car with a little time before the conference. She was anxious to tell Joe all the good news.

I am going to park the car and will stop up to see dad for a minute before we haul the Buick away. I will meet you in his room." Ted said.

"Your dad would like that, thanks."

Chapter 9 Prepare for Home

Ted walked in shortly after Sally got into Joe's room and noticed his dad trying to cut off the bandage from his hand with his table knife, which the nurse had wrapped around his hands to protect his IV. Sally was aghast as she asked. "What are you doing?"

"I must get this stuff off my hand because my hand really hurts. Hi Ted, it is nice of you to come to see me."

"Pops, what are you doing with that knife. You cannot be doing that."

" Sally could see he had an antibiotic but had stopped. When the nurse came in and unwrapped the hand and checked the site. It was swollen and very red and appeared to be infiltrated.

The nurse pulled the needle from his hand and wrapped warm towels around it and said to Joe. "No wonder your hand hurt the fluid went outside the vein, but it will feel much better now. I may have to restart your IV in your other arm, but the doctor just came in and was talking about starting you on oral antibiotics as you will be going home soon so I'm going to talk to him first. You may be in luck."

"Does this happen often, that's looks horrible?" Ted asked.

"Sometimes the IV needle gets disturbed and pulls slightly out of the vein and fluid goes into the surrounding tissue, which causes this. Your dad sometimes when he gets restless, he tends to pull on things he feels are not in a normal spot and irritates the area. He should be fine. Hopefully, the doctor will discontinue the IV and have him start his medications by mouth. This will also prepare him for going home." She explained sweetly.

Ted said to his dad, "Sounds like you are coming home soon. Won't that be nice."

" Great! Hallelujah and praise the Lord."

"You got that right, Pops. I must go now and am taking the Buick to fix it. I am bringing your old car for Sally to use, tomorrow."

"You are a good son, thanks. See you when I come home. Goodbye."

Ted hugged his dad and with tears in his eyes, left.

Sally went over to Joe hugged him and said, "That was nice of your son to come to see you. How are you doing? Have you been good to the staff?"

"I can't get into too much trouble, every time I try to sit up my bed buzzes."

"That is good you are not supposed to get up without their help

"The doctor came in a few minutes later and said to Joe, "Looks like you did an excellent job on helping us get your IV out of your arm. We are going to start you on antibiotics by mouth and get you home in three days. Which will be Thursday' How does that sound to you?'

"I cannot wait to get home and not have the buzzers going when I try and get out of bed. To look for my wife"

" You will not have to look for me. I may be looking for you. Maybe we should take the buzzers home to use?" Sally smiled

"No, I promise I will be good. I really will be going home on Thursday. Right doc?"

"Right, but you will have to not give your young wife any trouble or worry if you wander away, okay?"

"I won't, unless I forget," Joe said innocently.

"I will be in to see you a few times before you leave. Right now, the nurses and social service people will get you set up so you will have help at home, Thursday."

The gal from social service came in at that time and said, "Sounds like a good starting day. I will have his main nurse come and give him a little more time to orient to what Joe is expected to do and check out his environment on Friday. PT and OT will start Monday and Tuesday of next week. Nurses will come Wednesdays, Thursdays, and Fridays of each week. We made a list of each day and the hours when each different personnel will come, and we will give you a list of their schedules. I will notify Meal on wheels. They usually come three times a week around noon. After the nurses' visits."

"So, Thursday will be the pending day unless the unforeseen happens. We will have his medications given at 6 am and 12 noon on Thursday and we will send along enough of his antibiotic to give him at 6pm and 12midnight dose on Thursday and through the weekend to take 6am, 12 noon 6pm and 12am, Friday Saturday until Sunday at noon for last dose and then will be completed. All his other medications are the same as before. If something happens with his health care, just let his nurse know. He will notify the doctor or unless it is an emergency call 911. How does this sound, do you think you will be able to manage it? the nurse stated.

"I am a little in shock right now. I think I can manage Joe, but I do not know if I can manage myself asking for help. I always think I can. manage this job all by myself. Which I know is not always right. I always think I can figure it out on my own. I have a tough time asking for help, so I may need somebody to just ask me if I need help."

"I am sure your family will offer. They want to help your dad out also. Sometimes if you do not ask them for help. It may hurt them." The Gal from social services stated,

"You are right. That is something I will work on to not be such a mother hen. Lord will help me. Thanks for all the support for him, his family and for me. We appreciate it now and when we bring Joe home."

After the care plan was finished and they all left, Sally asked Joe," Do you understand that you will be going home on Thursday. That will be in three days?"

"Good. Hallelujah Praise the Lord. I'll be going home, and I don't think you're a mother hen." He said soberly.

Sally laughed as she remembered the words 'only a little child will see or know God.' Then she soberly reminded Joe, "When we take you home, remember nurses and others will be coming to our house to care for you during the week and on weekends your children will come more often. Won't that be nice?"

"I'd like that but where are you going?"

"Oh, I'll be there most of the time with you, but sometimes I will be getting groceries or do other chores while they are checking you."

"Will I be able to wear my britches and clothes?"

"Of course, we won't take those from you unless for bedtime, or you have to go back to hospital if you get sick again."

" I sure do not want to go there and be sick again. That was not fun."

"I know that was not fun for any of us. But we now know God gave us a miracle. And He will help you if you should get ill, again. Now you're able to go home."

"God is good. Hallelujah Praise the Lord."

"You know what? God gave us another miracle, yesterday. You know about my car problems with the dead battery? Well, your son took the Buick, and he is bringing our old car back tomorrow. Your daughter wanted a bigger car and didn't really like our little car. So, Ted is going to fix up the Buick for her and we will get out Nissen back. And it will be more dependable and easier to get around in."

"That nice. God is good. What else was wrong besides the battery' since Ted had to bring you here and haul the old car home?"

"Ted was not sure; the new battery was even dead this morning. But your angel of a son worked things out for us."

" What? my son, why do you call him an Angel?

"That's another story." Sally told Joe that after she prayed for help with her car, God told her in a dream that He was sending an Angel to help her. Then later, Ted came along and helped her with all she needed. So, Ted is our Angel. He is a wonderful man." Sally said with a smile which also made Joe smile.

"A wonderful man right, but an Angel, I'm not so sure. He's an Angel for helping you, though, I'll go for that," Joe said.

Sally thought to herself, sometimes Joe makes a lot more sense than a whole lot of people, without dementia.

Chapter 10 Another Sleepover

The two visited for some time when suddenly Sally realized it was too late for the city bus so she asked the nurse if she could sleep in Joes' reclining chair another night? I missed my bus to get home."

The nurse came in with Joe's dinner, she also brought in a tray for Sally and spoke. "It is nice you can stay. Being you will be by his side we can take his beeper off. You will hear him and be able to take him to the bathroom if he does wake up, right?"

"Oh, for sure. I can get practice to bring him home. He does well to get up, but I am always on alert that he makes it back to his bed without getting lost or falling."

"I am sure this must be trying on your family, "The nurse said with empathy.

"Right, seems like we are on a rollercoaster ride with his difficulties, but I know we have Jesus' riding alongside

"I love that! You are right. Jesus is with you. If you want, you can take Joe for a walk and have a cup of coffee in the lounge. He may like that. I will take his beeper off as long as you are with him."

"Good idea, Come on Joe, let's go for a walk and have a cup of coffee."

"Okey dory. I'm ready."

The two took a nice stroll to the patient lounge, Sally poured coffee and sat down with her husband, and they enjoyed the time together and occasionally watching TV. About an hour later, the nurse came in and told Joe. "We have some medications for you, and we will get you ready for bed and PT has exercises for you. Sally, you can wait here a little longer and finish your coffee. We will have your chair set up also for you."

"I will come back to your room, after you get all prettied up." Sally smiled.

That night Joe had a restful sleep, knowing his wife was by his side and the irritating IV was gone. Sally slept comfortably on the recliner. She didn't hear her husband any time until early the next morning

After eating breakfast with her husband, then while his caregivers kept Joe busy with his chores and PT and OT, Sally went to the lounge to make phone calls. She called for a city bus to come to the hospital. They would come in half an hour.

She then called Joe's daughter, Ann, and asked her if she would like to come with her to pick up her dad on Thursday. If you can come to our house around noon, I would like to take you out for lunch. Your dad will be busy with his care and the doctor will need to come in to check him, so we can pick him up at 2pm, together. I know your dad would appreciate it. He will feel comfortable knowing you are there to help him get settled."

"That would be good. I would love to help him. I will be there about noon, and lunch sounds great. I will need to be at work around 5pm. Thank you for asking."

After finishing the calls and coffee, she went back to Joe's room and giving her hubby a kiss, said. "I must catch my bus in a few minutes. I'll also get our car and do some shopping to get things ready for you to come home. I'll try to get in to see you tomorrow morning and on Thursday we'll be coming to take you home right after your lunch. Your daughter, Ann, will be coming with me to help get you settled when you are home. I love you."

"Love you too. I'll be waiting until you get back." Joe said.

When Sally finally got home on the bus, she ran in and saw her beautiful Nissan sitting in the garage with the car keys hanging in the key slot in the house.

She jumped into the familiar car and drove to pick up some groceries and a gate to put in front of the stairway.

Then she put her feet up to settle down for a while. She was exhausted after the final details of Joe's coming home in two days. She had to stock up on all the things and get things ready for him to come home. They had to put up the gate she got for the stairway, because Joe walked by there when he'd take his strolls around at night. She also had to remember to keep doors locked and remove hazards in the areas where he could fall. It was a process and trial getting ready to protect her hubby. It was sad to see him every day seem more like a child. Then a little voice came into her head, "Only as a little child will you be able to see God and know Him," Sally knew this message was from God. It eased her soul.

Sally knew this rollercoaster ride for them would be bumpy, but she was also assured that with God along, why should she worry? But her human nature of having to do it all by herself, always got in her own way. She prayed. " please God help me follow and obey your will and not mine. In Jesus name. Amen.

Chapter 11 Home at last

When Sally and Ann brought Joe home from the hospital. He was so excited and happy to be home. He just kept looking around and saying, "Is this my home? This is my home, right?"

"Yes, this is your home and you'll be here for a long time. You're going to have some people come over to help you while you're here. Nurses and other helpers will be here to check you out, take you for walks, and check your status and see how well you are doing."

"Can't you do all that as my nurse?"

"The nurses' will do it, that is their job, but I'll be here with you most of the time. I may be doing some chores while they're here. But will be done before they leave. Tomorrow your nurse a nice male nurse named Jay will be coming to check you and explain everything to you. You'll like him. How does this sound?"

" Okay, I'm just glad to get out of that other place. They had beepers and buzzers all around me all the time, besides all that they wouldn't even let me keep my britches on. You won't do that here will you?"

" No way. Sally won't take you britches away from you except when you go to bed." Ann said to her dad. I'm going to visit for a while but have to leave to get back to work at 4 tonight. You know I'm a working girl."

"I'm glad you came to visit and help get me home. I miss my children when you're not here."

" We miss you too dad when we aren't able to be with you. But your wife and your nurses will take care of you." Ann said. as she turned to wipe tears from her eyes

Remember tomorrow your nurse will be here so they'll keep you busy. He'll be checking your blood pressure and all your vital signs heart rate and also check out yours living place here so you will be safe. Then at the weekend I'll be here, and your children said they will be coming over more frequently. Like we talked about in the hospital." Sally said.

" That will be great. I love that when they come to visit, " Joe said.

He was very calm and understanding while visiting with his daughter. Sally thought, this is great, he seems like his old self.

After Ann was ready to leave, she gave her dad a kiss on his cheek and said, "Off to work I go, but I or one of your other children will come to see you Saturday or Sunday. Okay?"

" Okay. See you soon, don't forget me."

After Ann left, Sally fixed dinner and the two enjoyed a nice meal of Joe's favorite foods.

Joe said. "Wow that was a meal. I must be dreaming; I haven't had a meal like that for a long time."

"Thanks, I'm so happy to have you home. We thought we were going to lose you. But you proved you were strong, and we thank God that He showed His healing power."

After eating, the two sat and enjoyed reminiscing about all the blessings they had over the years. Joe seemed his normal self, both laughing at the different antics they had gone through over the almost 20 years of their wedded life.

Later they both readied for bed and as they crawled into their bed, Joe said, "It is so good to be home out of that other place, wherever that was. But now this is home. I can even be with my wife in my own bed."

"I'm also happy you're here with me." The two held hands and they both prayed a prayer of thanksgiving for all the blessing they had been given. Soon Joe was sound asleep.

Sally laid awake thinking how fast things changed in their lives, bringing back the memory of her mom when she was diagnosed with dementia after a stroke and broken hip and hospitalization, when she was in her early 80's.

Since her dad was not able to care for her, she was sent to a nursing home, and he was so lost without her.

Sally vowed she would try as long as she could without placing her hubby in a Long-Term Care unit. She was going to stay on this roller coaster ride knowing the Lord Jesus was with her.

She also recalled when her dad died about 4 years after his wife was placed in the home, the family took her out of the home for his funeral. They stood around their dads casket, all holding hands, as their mother said the Lord's prayer all the way through. When done she asked, "Now who was that dear man in the box?"

The family sadly, told her, "that was Teddy, your husband."

"Oh no, not my Teddy," she said and started crying. That was the first time she realized her husband of almost 70 years was gone and 6 months later she quit eating while in the nursing home and joined her Teddy in heaven.

Sally prayed quietly, "Please Lord, keep me on the right track and not let me give up as we travel through this long rollercoaster ride. I know it will be a rough ride, and I thank and trust you will be with us to get us through.

Chapter 12 Yo-Yo Hospital/ ER Trips

The next day, after a good sleep for both of them and after they had eaten breakfast, Joe's nurse, Jay, came over and visited with him. He checked his environment for safety and said, "I think you're in a safe home here. Now we'll check how well you are doing physically, "as he checked his heart, lungs and vital signs, Jay asked, "How are you feeling about being home again."

"I'm so happy to be out of that prison with all the buzzing and beeping around me."

Jay smiled and visited for a while longer while Sally was able to get chores done around the house she needed to do.

Saturday, Joe's children visited their dad while Sally went to refill Joe's medications and pick up items they needed.

The PT physical therapist came on Monday and took Joe for walks around the house to check his gait and steadiness and felt Joe was having slightly more difficulty. He was encouraged to use a cane or walker to prevent falls which he frequently was having.

The occupational therapist arrived on Tuesday to check his cognitive ability. A normal of 5 had lowered to 4 when he was diagnosed with dementia, about a month before he was hospitalized. After hospitalization his cognitive level went from 4 to 3.5 which showed deterioration of his ability to remember his surroundings and where he was and even starting to forget many names of people around him, he'd known most of his life. He often remembered his past when he was still living on the farm with his parents, but recent things he couldn't remember.

When home he remained steady at this level, for the three weeks he had home nurses. But when the nurses left, Joe would roam around the house calling out, " Mom, Dad? Where are you? I can't do anything anymore. My head is empty," he would say as he pounded his head. Seeing this, Sally knew he was suffering, and there was nothing she could do. She would take Joe's hands and cry out to God, "please help him find peace. Don't let him suffer, like this In Jesus name, Amen."

Joe would calm down and his attitude would change. So, whenever he would have these episodes, they would pray. This was several times, during his tough times. We made A daily habit of it. And put on his favorite music which always seemed to calm him.

After the three weeks end of nurses, March 2019 Sally took Joe to his doctor when he suddenly couldn't move both his arms, frozen like.

He was very uncomfortable, and the doctor told him after X rays, " You have bad arthritis and bone on bone apparently from a bad injury, which makes it difficult to move your arms. surgery is usually required, but with your conditions and age we feel that surgery would only cause more problems so we will try a cortisone shot to take down the swelling and start you on physical therapy to build and strength the muscles around the area. April 1st, 2019, he had his first Cortisone shot and with home PT he was able to get by and was good for a while. This was just the start of his yo-yo of hospital and ER trips .

Chapter 13 Lost Sense of Reality, but Calm

The year 0f 2020 Joe was progressing well physically, his mental cognitive level was 3.5 to 3 which caused crazy activities as if he'd be disassociated from reality. When he did these things, it would be so difficult he would become quite frustrated and angry at himself. It was difficult for Sally to see. She wasn't able to help him at these times.

One day he said to Sally, " my feet really hurt today." Sally checking his feet noticed he had his shoes on the wrong feet. Sally had to choke back laughing and said, " let's exchange the shoes and put each shoe on the other foot."

After helping him do just that he said, "you know what, my feet don't hurt anymore."

It was hard for Sally to see her husband becoming more and more like a little child as his cognitive levels decreased. She could sense that it would be harder and harder to care for him at home, but she had to hang in with him. And knowing God was with her, kept her going.

As his cognitive levels lowered his behavior and motor skills deteriorated.

Many times, Sally would see him try to put two legs into one pants leg or pull his pants on with his shoes on. That would have been quite an achievement, but it never worked. Sally had to tell him every time, "Joe, you must take your shoes off before putting your britches on."

Sally could see the frustration and fear in Joe's eyes, as he realized he was losing his sense of reality. He would always pound his head and say, " I can't do anything right, anymore. This head is empty." That had to be a horrible feeling as he tried doing his most simple chores. He was going up and down, up and down as if he was on a continual escalator and not getting anywhere.

He would sleep in his reclining chair at night, and one night he had to go to the bathroom, but Sally could not get him out of the chair. His strength was stronger than Sally's and he would pull her towards him, and suddenly she would be in his lap and couldn't get up until he let go. She finally just let him stay in the chair and he slept there all night, just like a baby. Next day he got up to the bathroom on his own. She never knew how he was able to do that. Sometimes he was perfectly normal and then completely raveled not knowing how to do things the next minute. That's why Sally always had to be on alert.

The worst thing Sally feared when he would wander about at night, that he would fall or go outside. He at times could figure how to get the outside door unlocked. Or at times while wandering ended up in a closet or got lost and couldn't remember how to get out of places. Sally was finally able to encourage him to always use his cane or walker when he got up. She then could hear his tap-tap-tap on the floor and she was able to be on the alert.

Sally knew how tragic this had to be for him; not knowing where to go or where he was As it was also tragic for Sally as she didn't know what to expect next.

Somedays, Sally would cry out to God, "I just can't do this anymore."

Then that voice she always recognized, answers, "I'm on the roller coaster ride with you. Hang in there, I won't let you or hubby ever fall down that cliff."

This would remind her, and things would go nicely for a while and some days perfectly. And then other days, not so. And she again remember God was with always with them.

Many days if Sally had to run on errands, she would have to take her hubby and they would casually stop at a restaurant. It would be difficult as many times she'd have to get others to help her get him out of his chair. They started using a wheelchair he could stay in, worked much better when Sally took him place's. One day Sally took him along with her to a place which they had enjoyed many times before he got sick. He enjoyed it at first and with his short attention span got restless and he wheeled away, and she had to look for him and caught him almost trying to get out the emergency door.

That put a caboose on most adventures they could have together. Church was not attempted at all as his cognitive levels dropped. He would get so restless and disturb others or suddenly he couldn't move and just stare as if he was having a seizure. It was dramatic as if he was having a stroke which was becoming more frequent. Sally was fearful for him and the rest of the church members that he would do something unusual.

Sally decided it was easier and she could get help faster if they just stayed home.

But feeling their need for church, the two would sit and watch 4 hours of TV evangelism, that way if Joe's attention span shortened, he could get up and walk around as needed. But surprisingly when he was home, he really enjoyed and loved just listening to God's word, and the church music. Since he loved church music, this became his tranquillizer, even when they weren't watching TV or if he became restless the music would calm him down and he became very content.

Then many times Joe would say he wanted to go home. Sally didn't understand at first that his real home he wanted to go to be his home with his Jesus in heaven. When Sally realized what home, her Joe was talking about, they decided they both needed to use more time together talking with Jesus.

Sally knew Joe was a child of God, and happy he would be in heaven when he died. She said, " I know you want to be with Jesus in heaven and I believe you will be, but I believe also he has plans here on earth for you, before you will be with Him."

" Yes, I am concerned for my children to come to know and love Jesus as I do. I should be Praying more for them. Maybe that's what God is waiting for."

"That could be, so let us pray for them right now to come to know how great God is."

The two sat holding hands and prayed for all their children to know and ask Jesus into their hearts. And every day that was their prayer together.

This was a time Sally and Joe would sit and were able to talk and laugh and even sing songs together. They would tell jokes and talk about the old days and surprisingly Joe could remember the old days much better than yesterday. He would tell Sally about the funny things he did. Sally wasn't sure if he was making these things up or normally happened, but she enjoyed his openness at the time. Then all of a sudden, he'd talk about something strangely different.

But Sally would think to herself." Well, that's my Joe, may as well get used to these weird changes." And she was able to go along with many things he'd say or do, and they could laugh together.

Sally was also thinking that Joe may be feeling that she was more in line with his cognitive level. That was okay with Sally as she was starting to see and believe that God was giving this time together to prepare them both for the inevitable future.

Joe was having an increase in little strokes which she knew would cause his cognitive levels to edge closer down to 2, where he may be completely dependent on her or others without having these times of togetherness.

Then in May 2020, tragedy again hit their family, when Sally's youngest and Joe's stepson passed away suddenly in his sleep from a blood clot. He was also a buddy to Joe. The two would sit for hours talking and smoking on their front porch.

Sally could see that Joe was also grieving along with her.

Sally, even while grieving, felt she had to take the responsibility of making preparations for his funeral, since he didn't have a wife or significate other. "Please God help me with this. I don't even know how to start. I Certainly don't have money for a funeral."

Then Sally's other sons came to her rescue and took over all the details and between them all paid for his funeral costs, as he did not have insurance. This was a gift from God and Sally was so thankful to God and her family.

One of his daughters was able to come and be with her dad so he wouldn't be left alone when she talked with the other people.

Joe did well at the funeral as long as he was with his daughter, but he wasn't able to visit with others as he didn't know anyone except Sally's family. He didn't even realize who had died. He just knew there was a funeral. That was hard on Sally, but she was thankful for his daughter to be with him. Since it was during covid, they didn't have a very long funeral and no lunch was served. Many of their old neighbors, relatives and friends came to give their condolences, which helped the family get through.

When the year 2021 came along, it was very difficult to go anywhere with Sally's joe. His attention span was so short, he would love an adventure and suddenly hate it for no real reason.

Fourth of July 2021 was one example when the family went on a pontoon ride touring a large lake and Joe was really enjoying it when suddenly he got up and walked to edge of pontoon saying, "I need to get off, " our sons had to stop him from jumping into the lake.

They all finally encouraged him to sit down beside Sally, as she hugged him and told him they would get him off safely. Then the family quickly turned the pontoon around and headed home at a rapid pace. When they got to the dock, It took four strong men to get him off the pontoon and up the dock to the land.

Sally knew he had always had a fear of being in water, but loved being on boats. She was puzzled by the great fear he suddenly had. Once he was on land and sitting in his wheelchair, he was content.

This was just another excursion they had to scratch off their short itinerary, but Sally knew that God was with them once again

Chapter 14 Continual Downhill Spiral

The year 2021 continued slowly and also Joe's cognitive levels were slowly heading to the 2 Level. Sally knew that his time was getting close to when she wouldn't be able to take care of him much longer by herself.

One day when Joe went to the doctor for another checkup the doctor could see his cognitive decline. He asked him, "Who are you living with now?"

He answered, "My mom and dad, my brother (all which have died several years ago) and my two kids. No wife was mentioned. Sally was a little hurt by this, but she understood his situation.

The doctor asked Sally, "How really are things going at home?"

Sally truthfully said, "Not good. He doesn't remember who I am. I'm terrible afraid of his roaming at night. He got lost in the closet one night. When I asked him to come sleep in our bed so I could hear him, he said. 'I can't we're not married.' When I asked who I was he said, 'my nurse.' He apparently has morals, and I must be doing something right as his nurse," Sally said laughing.

The doctor laughed and asked Joe. "who is this young lady sitting here beside you?"

Joe looked over at Sally and said innocently, " If she's a young lady she can't be my wife. I'm too old for her. I think she's my nurse as she's been taking care of me."

The doctor said, "Let me tell you a little secret, just between you and me. She may be a young lady, but she is your wife."

Joe looked over at Sally and said, "Are you really my wife? Oh, I knew that."

The doctor asked Sally, after the nurse took Joe for blood tests. "Does Joe try to hurt you at home and are you safe?"

"Oh no, he's never raised a hand to me. He' very docile. He gets more angry at himself; he keeps punching his head saying he doesn't have anything inside there he doesn't know what he's doing at all. It's strange, sometimes he is so normal, and he doesn't have anything that he says or seems weird and then within seconds, he will be completely talking irrationally. He's really hard to understand how to take him and what to do with him. Lately we have been able to communicate, I sometimes act dumb, or act confused myself, which I feel seems to help us relate better and laugh and joke with each other. We even sang together, prayed together and talked about different things. He loves to talk about his farm life and some dumb things he used to do. He sounded so normal. Sometimes I think he was making some of that up, I wasn't sure, but it seemed normal to him. Then the next second It was like he would just sit and stare and then shake and punch his head and then say something strange, which was really weird, and this has been going on for several months."

"Are you able to get household duties done? The doctor asked

"Yes and no. I've been trying to work outside to get a few things done out in the backyard. I would ask him to come out and help. Occasionally he would and then suddenly he'd be gone and usually go back indoors, but one day when I thought he had gone inside, I heard a car out in the front yard I ran to the front and our car was sitting halfway out of the driveway. He apparently realized he couldn't drive with no driver's license, so he went over to the neighbors to help him find his wife. Not seeing me, she called the police.

When I noticed that he was at the neighbors, I asked him, what he was doing? "I was looking for you where were you?"

I told him where I was. The neighbor sheepishly told me she called the cops. l told her that's good. I can explain to them, if my husband gets lost or ends up walking away and I don't notice, he'll know where to bring him home. These are the things which are what I'm a little fearful of."

The doctor said, "You certainly have a lot on your plate. We will try to get some help to give you some relief. Does his children help and take him very much?"

Sally said, "They take them when they can. But I think they have a tough time doing that, because he has wandered away and they had to go look for him. They have 10 acres, so he'd be hard to find. They come when they can but they're awfully busy and I don't really want them to have to run over every time Joe has a problem. His son came over when he fell and helped him a lot and they've helped us with getting a different car and they were really good that way. And his daughters call and come when they can. Sometimes he doesn't know them, so they have a tough time coming around, that has to be scary to see him that way."

"Maybe daycare would work, and he could feel like he's doing something practical."

"That would be great. He wants to chop wood or milk cows. This could be his 'job,' Sally said.

The doctor then said, "Okay that would be the plan. I'll have Social Services call you and you can collaborate with them or maybe get him in Adult Daycare's Program. That should give you some relief. Joe is definitely declining in his cognitive level and someday pretty soon he won't be able to do anything for himself so you will need much more help in the future. Is he starting to need help with any of his own hygiene cares?"

"I've been helping to get him in the tub and make sure he is dressed properly. He put things on backwards shoes on the wrong feet and different things. I usually try to explain to him how to do it and he's OK with it until the next time he does it. It is a repetitive thing. I have to keep reminding him and to be honest, I'm getting exhausted, and I don't know what else I can do. Maybe having daycare for a while would just give me a little break so I can get the house cleaned and do things around the house and finish my yard work I need to get done that would be a great relief."

"OK we'll get working on that and the social service will be calling you and letting you know all about finances and what to expect. Joe seems to be doing fairly well physically. His mental health will be our primary project for both your sakes." When the nurse came back, they packed up their things. Joe said, "Thanks Doc for all your help and I'll take my wife, I think, home." they all had a good laugh.

Chapter 15 'Job' at Adult Daycare

Social service notified Sally the next week and told Sally, "Joe qualifies for an Adult Day Care program in the city. He will start next Monday morning. A nurse from the center will call you in about an hour to give you the details of what to expect. His nurse will be Amy."

Amy called an hour later and said, "We are anxious to have Joe visit our facility.

We are proud of what to offer. We will have a bus at your house in t h e mornings to pick him up at 7: 30 so he will be here by 8 am. There will be other passengers with similar problems, so he will not feel out of place. They will give him a breakfast snack and lunch around 1 pm.

They have games and many activities and necessary needs of their daily hygiene habits and cleanliness is observed and helped encouraged as needed.

Then we have them all pick anything they have worked on be put away and any gear put in its proper place. They are then ready and wait for their bus to come. Some need more help than others to get on. If Joe needs walker, a cane or wheelchair bring yours and we will label it and make sure it gets home with them. If you would like to bring him in and he can get adjusted to the environment."

I think that would be a good idea. He thinks he is going to a job, and thinks he should drive. So, I will bring him Monday and you can bring him home at 2."

"Okay, see you Monday around 8 am."

"Joe was surprisingly dressed in his apparel all on the proper way and shoes even on the right feet. He looked so handsome and normal, she even forgot he had a problem.

They had a quick breakfast and took off, Sally driving. When they got to his "job: Sally walked in with, and they were introduced to the other clients and personnel. They were all so friendly Joe joined right in, barely saying goodbye.

The first day when Joe came home on the bus, he came over to Sally and hugged her and excitedly said? "I love you; I love you. But I have a new girlfriend."

"That's nice. More power to you, You must have had an enjoyable time." Sally smiled and gave him a kiss. He was really good when he went to daycare,

That week went fairly well for the first few days, but he wouldn't always get on the bus in the morning, he didn't think he had to take a bus he wanted to drive to his 'job,' so Sally convinced him that she would take him in the morning, but he had to come home on the bus.

This worked out for a while, but the last day he was in the Daycare of that week, when they brought him home, he couldn't or wouldn't move to get off the bus. It was as if he was having a seizure or a small stroke.

The driver was frustrated he didn't know what to do. He said, " You have to get off now. I have to get others home to their families."

Sally tried and couldn't get him off even with two people helping, he stood there stoically and just stared ahead. Nobody could get him to do anything, so the bus driver had to call the police.

Sally had finally coaxed him to get off the bus and by the time the police got there, he was in the house sitting at the table as if nothing had happened.

The first thing he said to the policeperson was, "Look what she did to me," as he pointed to his arm which was all swollen and bruised from an area where he had slammed his hand in a door, several weeks earlier.

Sally stood back and was shaking as she said, " I don't think you understand." As she tried to explain what happened.

"I understand," the policeperson said. "I know you didn't do this."

The policeperson explained to Joe. "You should not tell things about your wife. That aren't true. Your wife only wants to help you."

Apparently coming from the authorities, he understood and told Sally. "I'm sorry."

Sally said, "we need to call an ambulance. I believe my husband had a small stroke again and needs care"

The policeman called the ambulance and when they came it took the policeman, the two medics, Sally and her son to get Joe on the cart to go by ambulance to the hospital. Sally believes he thought that he was scared that he was going to have to go to jail. We all tried to explain to him he was going to see his doctor in the hospital to check him out.

Sally kissed him as he kept holding on to her as if he would lose her. Sally said, "I will meet you at the hospital."

When they finally settled him down and, in the ambulance, they took off with the lights sirens blazing. Tears fell from Sallys eyes as she knew she would not be caring for at home. He wouldn't be coming home again.

Sally went into the house washed the tears stains from her face and her son drove her to the hospital to be with her husband again in another emergency.

While sitting in ER waiting for word of her husband's condition. Sally's thoughts were of the good times they had together. She was positive that these times, through all the turning and twisting on their ride, God had given them to her for just a time as this. Sally then called his children about his situation. Most came just as the doctor walked in and said almost tearfully. to them, " Your dad is having repeated small strokes and has for some time. We believe that he is in his last stage of Dementia which is total care. He will not be able to be cared for at his home. Social Service is again looking for a permanent placement in a Memory Care Unit. His time will be short, so I suggest you all try to spend as much time with him as you can. Social services will keep in contact, and we will keep Joe here in the hospital until we find a nice place for him. He will have a week before his insurance for hospital care will run out. I'm sure something will come up."

Weeping was heard around the room. Sally, weeping herself, told Joe's children," This is not the end we still have him. We were just talking a few days how he wanted so much to be at home with his Jesus and he wanted you to all be by his side before he would leave to be with Jesus. His biggest fear he expressed to me is he wanted all his children to know, believe in Him and take Jesus into your hearts, so someday you shall meet again. These were his prayers for you.

Sally grieved for Joe but was happy about what his future would be and to look forward to, because he knew the Lord and was born again. That was such a consolation and help for Sally and his family.

Chapter 16 Joes New Home

The next day the social services called Sally and said that they had found a nice home with a memory care unit for him. We have a few things to go over with you and if you want to see the place, we can meet you there tomorrow morning at 10, and you can check it out then and meet its nurses and staff. Then if you like it there, we will be able to get him in toward the end of this week. I think your husband would like this home. It is at the edge of town, in the country, with a barn across the street. He will be having a roommate but he's fairly quiet and has very few visitors. They may be company for each other. The place is called, "A Home in the Country" on highway 61, just before the bridge going into Rush city. You will see a big sign along the road, with the name on it. See you there."

"That sounds great. I will ask his daughters to join me if they are able. See you tomorrow at 10am."

Sally was happy to hear the good news, as she was getting worried because the hospital may have to release him soon as his time of stay was over at the end of the week. She would either have to bring him home or pay for the extra stay. She knew she could not do either. But when she prayed about it, God answered her prayers again.

The next morning Joe's sisters came to her house, and they rode to the Home together. They loved the place as Sally also did. The final transaction was signed, and Joe was to be transferred by hospital bus in two days, one day short of his allowed time.

When Sally met Joe at his new home, he was sitting up in the chair joking with his nurses. He appeared to be comfortable. When his daughters and Sally arrived, he was happy to see them and said, "Here comes my family I knew they would come to my new home."

Sally was surprised he seemed to be so normal and very relaxed there. He knew he was at a place where he could feel comfortable and safe.

Sally would visit every day and his children would come and visit, at the weekend.

Then suddenly Joe regressed, and it became difficult for him to communicate. As he regressed, it was harder for them to come as he couldn't respond to them or anyone. He was unable to do anything for himself. And was difficult for his children to see.

The nurses would have to use a lift to get him out of bed, to put him in a chair to keep him from bedsores, because he was not able to do anything on his own. He was completely incapacitated.

He had not spoken for 2-3 days, when suddenly out if the blue as the nurses were placing him on the lift he said to the nurses, "do you know what you are doing?" The nurses were all stunned. After that he never spoke again.

Joe was going downhill fast. He refused to eat, and his body started to shut down and on Wednesday that first week, he was placed in hospice. His sister and her friend joined Sally, the day he was placed in hospice.

Sally would come in every day to see Joe. It was hard to see him deteriorate so fast. Sally came in later on Friday of that week and when she walked in immediately, she could see that Joe's system was failing. He had not been eating and was completely unable to respond to any reflexes.

The Hospice nurse told Sally when she arrived. "You better call his family. He's not going to make it much longer."

When Sally called the family one daughter told her, "They were not coming often because they figured he'd be there for a while, and they could come anytime.

The one daughter was planning to come that night but changed her mind and would come the next morning, with her sister. Sally tried to convince them by telling them, "The nurse feels you should come in tonight." When they couldn't come, Sally started to cry and handed the phone to the nurse and said, " You convince them to come."

The Hospice nurse took the phone and said, "This is the Hospice nurse. We feel you need to come right away; your dad's body is shutting down and will not make it through the night. In fact, he probably won't make it for more than two, three hours. You should come right away."

Well, within an hour, they were all there. The whole family that could make it. Sally was so thankful they all came. because one hour later. Their dad was gone. They were glad to be able to say their goodbyes. He wasn't responsive to them, but he knew they were there. And they prayed, laughed together and talked about the old times while he was there with them. When her dad was gone, his oldest daughter hugged Sally and said, " I'm glad you made us come in. We were able to see our dad leave, quietly, peacefully, as he went to be with his Jesus, with a smile on his face. "

This is not the end of this story because many people were and have since been blessed and also came to know Jesus

This will be the new beginning for Joe in heaven. We believe he is having the time of his life in his afterlife.

A Prayer for all who may be inflicted with this deadly disease and their family and caregivers. Remember that God will help you get through this rough time. Just keep holding onto His hands and He will lead you the right way.

Heavens Gained Another Angel

My face forgot how to smile.

My eyes forgot clarity and my

Breaths forgot steadiness for a while.

My mind forgets that it's not a forever goodbye.

My guarding heart, however, has no such fault

So ,it keeps a smile, a laugh, and a face

Stored deep within Mind's armored vault.

Memories are made for Time to erase,

So, it wasn't your fault that steadfast Time

Called a name and that the name was you.

I hope you remember, in the realm of the divine,

That love reaches beyond the grave and through

The ever-rotting, rusted chains of our mortal frames.

Your vault in me is here to stay, until I too meet Time's decay.

I remember that last day on the docks of Adley.

Together we watched the waves as you gladly

offered me a cheerful "God bless you!"

Proving that your heart was still true.

Despite Time's powerful corruption,

Your heart was not part of that destruction

Now God is blessing you with perfect wings

And I have to fight against my heart's tears,

Because there, your one true life begins.

Now you are blessed to live above all fears

And likewise blessed, will I one day be.

For now, I'll miss what was and cherish what is,

Until the end finds me and I too am made free.

One day, we'll both wander the realm that is His.

Please save a smile as you fly through the clouds.

We will share it again when worldly chains

are broken and time has no more bounds.

We'll meet again at the gate between domains.

Poem by Bethy Kalpin written in the memory of the only grandpa on her dad's side, she had known.

In loving memory of James "Jim" Olson a loving husband. Father and grandfather.

I. NDEX: WHAT IS DEMENTIA

A. Dementia vs. Alzheimer's

1. What is the Difference?

comparison

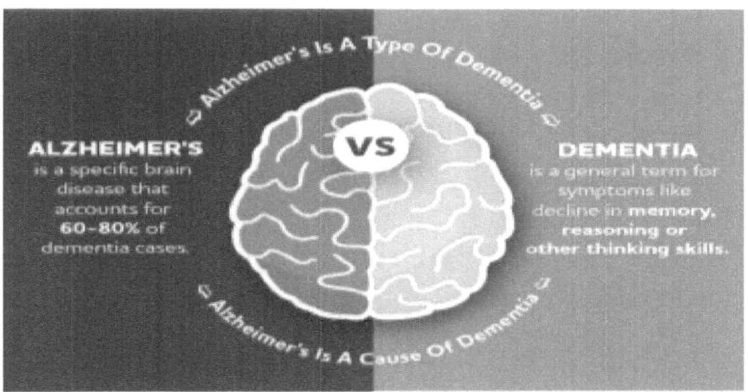

Dementia is a general term for a decline in mental ability severe enough to interfere with daily life, while Alzheimer's is a specific disease. Alzheimer's is the most common cause of dementia. Learning about the two terms and the difference between them is important and can empower individuals living with Alzheimer's or another dementia, their families and their caregivers with necessary knowledge.

2. Dementia Overview

Dementia describes a group associated with a decline in memory, reasoning or other thinking skills. Many different and many conditions cause the condition in which brain changes of more than one type of dementia occur simultaneously. Alzheimer's disease is the most common cause of dementia, accounting for 60-80% of dementia cases. Dementia is not a normal part of aging. It is caused by damage to brain cells that affects their ability to communicate, which can affect thinking, behavior and feelings. Dementia is a general term for loss of memory, which are severe language, problem-solving another thinking abilities enough to interfere with daily life. Alzheimer's is the most common cause of dementia. dementia is not a single disease, but an overall term to describe a collection of symptoms that one may experience if one is living with a variety of diseases, including Alzheimer's disease. Diseases grouped under the general term "dementia" are caused by abnormal brain changes. Dementia symptoms trigger a decline in thinking skills, also known as cognitive abilities, severe enough to impair daily life and independent function. They also affect behavior, and relationships. Alzheimer's is a progressive brain disease. This means the disease and resulting symptoms **worsen** over time. The disease often progress in 7 stages.

B. Seven Stages and Cognitive Levels.

Stage 1 _ Level 5 normal functioning, Normal. Some forgetfulness.

Stage2—Level 5-4.5, loses familiar objects unable to recall loved ones names

Stage 3—Level 4.5-4, gets lost while driving forgets birthdays or appointments

Stage 4 --Level 4-3.5, withdrawals socially, struggles with everyday tasks.

Stage 5—-Level3.5-3 forgets information or events. may wander and get lost in own home. Losing sense of Reality.

Stage 6—-Level 3-2.requires assistance with normal self-cares, and pronounce memory loss and loved one's names or who they are, Occasionally becomes abusive to strangers if he feels he is being forced and fearful of going to jail.

Stage 7—-Level 2—poor condition, debilitated, coordination affecting ability to walk or eat, impaired body functions.

C. Common Types of Dementias

1.**Alzheimers** most common- shrinkage of brain causes significate affects every brain functions causing many changed, particularly in behavior and interpersonal relationships

2. **Dementia with Lewy Bodies** also known "Cortical Lewy body disease" or " diffuse Lewy body disease" it's similar to Alzheimer's in that it can cause tremors and stiffness. May be accompanied with sleep disorders and visual hallucinations.

3.**Vascular Dementia**-also referred as "muti-infarction" or "poststroke dementia" strokes and vascular accidents causing tissue loss and brain damage causing memory 1 wrong decision making, and difficulty in planning

4.**Frontotemporal Dementia-** neurodegeneration affects frontal and temporal lobes in brain and personality emotional and cognitive impairment.

5.**Mixed Dementia** when someone is affected by 2 types of dementia. The brain changes into more than one type. Parkinson's disease may be considered part of this group.

D. Diagnostic Measures

To diagnose the cause of dementia, a health care professional must recognize the pattern of loss of skills and function. The care professional also determines what the person is still able to do. More recently, biomarkers have become available to make a more accurate diagnosis of Alzheimer's disease. A health care professional reviews your medical history and symptoms and conducts a physical exam. Someone who is close to you may be asked about your symptoms as well. No single test can diagnose dementia. You'll likely need a number of tests that can help pinpoint the problem.

<u>a. Cognitive and neuropsychological tests</u>

These tests evaluate your thinking ability. A number of tests measure thinking skills, such as memory, orientation, reasoning and judgment, language skills, and attention.

<u>b. Neurological evaluation</u>

Your memory, language skills, visual perception, attention, problem-solving skills, movement, senses, balance, reflexes and other areas are evaluated.

<u>c. Brain Tests</u>

CT or MRI. These scans can check for evidence of stroke, bleeding, tumor or fluid buildup, known as hydrocephalus.

PET scans. These scans can show patterns of brain activity. They can determine whether amyloid or tau protein, hallmarks of Alzheimer's disease, have been deposited in the brain.

<u>d. Laboratory tests</u>

Simple blood tests can detect physical problems that can affect brain function, such as too little vitamin B-12 in the body or an underactive thyroid gland. Sometimes the spinal fluid is examined for infection, for inflammation or for markers of some degenerative diseases.

<u>e. Psychological Evaluation</u>

A mental health professional can determine whether depression or another mental health condition is contributing to your symptoms. Cognitive levels of Dementia ranging from 5normal- 2 complete need of care. The dimensions of cognitive ability in dementia have been studied by researchers. Principal components analysis of neuropsychological test scores for the dementia patients yielded the following 6 components:

(1) Memory/Learning, (2) Spatial/Nonverbal,

(3) Verbal/Lexical Knowledge,

(4) Verbal Fluency,(5) Visual Paired Associates(

6) Verbal Attention s In

<u>f. Check for Medicines </u>**(which may increase symptoms)**

<u>Benzodiazepines</u>, used to treat conditions such as anxiety, seizures and sleep disturbances

<u>Anticholinergics,</u> which affect chemicals in the nervous system to treat many diverse types of conditions

<u>Antihistamines</u>, often used to manage allergy symptoms

<u>Opioids</u>, often used to treat pain

<u>Proton pump inhibitors</u>, often used to treat reflux or gastro-esophageal reflux disease (Gerd)

Talk about your options with your doctor When thinking about any treatment, it is important to have a conversation with a health care professional to determine whether it is appropriate. A doctor who is experienced in using these medications should monitor people who are taking them and provide information that can help

E. Navigating Treatment Options

There is exciting progress in Alzheimer's and dementia research that is creating promising new treatments for people living with the disease. It is important to learn as much as you can about which drugs are available. Talk about your options with your doctor.

Your doctor may have a conversation with you about how well some of the Alzheimer's treatments work. They may discuss if the potential benefits outweigh the risk of any side effects. Taking a drug is a personal decision that each individual must make on their own with the help of doctors. You may want to ask your doctor.—Two different effects of drugs used:

1.Drugs that temporarily ease some symptoms of Alzheimer's disease.

2. Drugs that change disease progression in people living with Alzheimer's.

When thinking about any treatment, it is important to have a conversation with a health care professional to determine whether it is appropriate. Drugs in this category slow disease progression. They slow the decline of memory and thinking, as well as function, in people living with Alzheimer's disease.

<u>Aducanumab (Aduhelm®)</u> is an anti-amyloid antibody intravenous (IV) infusion therapy that is delivered every month. It has received accelerated

approval from the FDA to treat early Alzheimer's disease, including people living with mild cognitive impairment (MCI) or mild dementia due to Alzheimer's disease have confirmation of elevated beta-amyloid in the brain.

<u>Lecanemab (Leqembi®)</u> related reactions, amyloid-related imaging abnormalities (ARIA) and headaches. There is exciting progress in Alzheimer's and dementia research that is creating promising new treatments for people living with the disease. It is important to learn as much as you can about which drugs are available. Talk about your options with your doctor When thinking about any treatment, it is important to have a conversation with a health care professional to determine whether it is appropriate. A doctor who is experienced in using these medications should monitor people who are taking them and provide information that can help

1.Treatment Benefits and Side Effects

Your doctor may have a conversation with you about how well some of the Alzheimer's treatments work. They may discuss if the potential benefits outweigh the risk of any side effects. Taking a drug is a personal

decisions that each individual must make on their own with the help of doctors. You may want to ask your doctor: As Alzheimer's progresses, brain cells die a noncognitive connections among cells are lost. This causes cognitive (memory and thinking) and (behavioral and psychological) symptoms to worsen. While these medications do not stop the damage Alzheimer's causes to brain cells, they may help lessen or stabilize symptoms for a limited time.

Drugs in this category slow disease progression. They slow the decline of memory and thinking, as well as function, in people living with Alzheimer's disease.

Aducanumab (Aduhelm®) is an anti-amyloid antibody intravenous (IV) infusion therapy that is delivered every month. It has received accelerated approval from the FDA to treat early Alzheimer's disease, including people living with mild cognitive impairment (MCI) or mild dementia due to Alzheimer's disease who have confirmation of elevated beta-amyloid in the brain.

Aducanumab was the first therapy to demonstrate that removing beta-amyloid from the brain reduces cognitive and functional decline in people living with early Alzheimer's. The most common side effects are amyloid-related imaging abnormalities (ARIA), headache and fall.

Lecanemab (Leqembi®) is an anti-amyloid antibody intravenous (IV) infusion therapy that is delivered every two weeks. It has received traditional approval from the FDA to treat early Alzheimer's disease, including people living with mild cognitive impairment (MCI) or mild dementia due to Alzheimer's disease who have confirmation of elevated beta-amyloid in the brain.

Lecanemab was the second therapy to demonstrate that removing beta-amyloid from the brain reduces cognitive and functional decline in people living with early Alzheimer's. The most common reported side effects were infusion-related reactions, amyloid-related imaging abnormalities (ARIA) and headaches. There is exciting progress in Alzheimer's and dementia research that is creating promising new treatments for people living with the disease. It is important to learn as much as you can about which drugs are available. Talk about your options with your doctor When thinking about any treatment, it is important to have a conversation with a health care professional to determine whether it is appropriate. A doctor who is experienced in using these medications should monitor people who are taking them and provide information.

F. Words From the Author

I share this as I have lived with a wonderful person who was diagnosed with deadly dementia. He fought it for several years, and every year, it became more exhausting as if we were on a rollercoaster with no end in sight. He became almost like a child. When I would get frustrated, God would remind me in Mark 10:15 NIV Bible. 'I tell you the truth, anyone who will not receive the kingdom of God like a little child will never enter it.' this was always a comfort? Because when Joe would say continuously that he wanted to go home, I knew that he had that child-like love of God he knew as a little child. His home he wanted was to be with his Jesus.

Then in November 2021, after a short bout in hospital and unable to come home he was placed in a wonderful and caring memory care unit for seven days, and with all his family present, 8*-year-old Joe was taken home to be with His Jesus, which was his prayer. He is now whole, and I'm sure loving his new home. But he is missed here on earth.

Never give up on your loved one, even though you feel as if you're on a rollercoaster ride. Just ask Jesus to help you, and He will ride with you. Be kind and love them even if they don't know you and think we are their Mom or nurse. I know, God has a special place for them, and some day we may see them again.

G. References and Resources

1.The Mayo Clinic

https://wwwmayoclinic.org/

2. NIH National Institute on aging

Https://www.nia.nih.gov/health/[1]

3.Alzheimer's Organizations.

https://www.alz.org/

Research continuing at many Mayo Clinics, and

Alzheimer's Organization's, In search of a cure. God Bless all for your dedication to try to find a cure

There is exciting progress in Alzheimer's and dementia research that is creating promising new treatments for people living with the disease. It is important to learn as much as you can about which drug is the best and safest drug to use.

---

1. https://www.nia.nih.gov/health/

H. Other Books by Author

1.<u>The Truth shall set you Free</u> (A young n life of abuse, flees her abusers in search of freedom.

2.<u>Train Wreck in the Sierras</u> (An elderly couple, the only survivor of a Terrorist, flee for their lives as they know too much.

3.<u>Life After</u> <u>Death.</u> A family's walk in the shadow of a loved one's suicide. (2- book series next)

4.<u>Bitter Betrayal, but Sweet is Revenge</u> (Revenge is not always sweet, and forgiveness and love is.)

5.<u>Oh No, My Ex is Back</u>()And causing trouble Again.)

6.<u>Terror in Texas.</u> (A Mexican gang inflicts fear, pain and suffering on an American family)

7.<u>Story of Kaylee's Young Life, Though the Eyes of Her Granny.</u> (When snakes enters Kaylee's yard, one day Granny, seeing her fear and curiosity, explained why and how sin and fear of snakes came into the world.

1.Bible Verses for Hope and Encouragement

<u>Mark 10:15 NIV Bible.</u> 'I tell you the truth, anyone who will not receive the kingdom of God like a little child will never enter it.

<u>Matthew 11:28,29,30</u>

28 "Come onto me, all who labor and are heavy laden. And I will give you a rest.

29. Take My yoke upon you and you can learn from Me, for I am gentle and lowly in heart. And you will find rest for your souls.

30 . For my yoke is easy and my burden is light." Says the Lord.

<u>John 3:16,</u>

For God so loved the world, that he gave his only son that whosoever believes in Him shall not perish but have eternal life.

9 798224 988150

Acknowledgements

I am immensely grateful for the journey that "Unexpected Romance in Rio" has taken me on, and I extend my heartfelt thanks to everyone who has contributed to this unforgettable tale.

First and foremost, I express my deepest gratitude to Carlos and Isabela, whose vibrant personalities and captivating love story inspired the pages of this book. Your courage, resilience, and unwavering belief in love have touched the hearts of readers around the world.

I am indebted to the colorful tapestry of Rio de Janeiro's Carnival, which served as the perfect backdrop for Carlos and Isabela's journey. The pulsating energy, the lively music, and the rich culture of Brazil infused every chapter with a sense of celebration and joy.

To the readers who have embarked on this adventure with Carlos and Isabela, thank you for your enthusiasm, your feedback, and your unwavering support. Your presence has made this journey even more meaningful, and I hope that their story has resonated with you in profound ways.

A special mention goes to the characters who brought depth and complexity to the narrative—each one contributing a unique perspective and adding layers of intrigue and emotion to the story.

I extend my gratitude to my family and friends for their encouragement, patience, and understanding throughout the writing process. Your love and belief in me have been a constant source of strength.

To my editors, designers, and everyone involved in bringing this book to life, thank you for your dedication, creativity, and expertise.

Your contributions have made "Unexpected Romance in Rio" a work of art that I am proud to share with the world.

Last but not least, I acknowledge the power of love itself—the force that drives us, inspires us, and reminds us of the beauty of human connection. May we always find joy, passion, and unexpected moments of romance in our own lives.

With gratitude and love,
Mikey Katodiya

Prologue

In the heart of Rio de Janeiro, where the rhythm of samba echoes through the streets and the vibrant colors of Carnival paint the sky, a love story unfolds like a symphony of emotions and experiences. This is the tale of Carlos and Isabela, two souls destined to cross paths amidst the enchanting chaos of Brazil's most celebrated festival.

As the sun sets on the city, casting a golden glow over the bustling crowds and lively music, Carlos finds himself drawn to the energy of Carnival. Little does he know that this night will change his life forever. Meanwhile, Isabela, with her infectious laughter and free spirit, navigates the festivities with a sense of wonder and curiosity.

Their paths converge in a moment of serendipity, a "First Glance at Carnival," where eyes meet and hearts begin to beat in synchrony. From that fleeting moment, a bond is forged—a connection that transcends the ordinary and ventures into the realm of destiny.

Through "Echoes of Laughter and Music," their story unfolds like a melody, each laugh and note carrying the promise of something magical. In "Whispers of the Heart," whispered confessions and shared dreams lay the foundation for a love that knows no bounds, a love that defies logic and reason.

"Dancing Under the Stars" becomes a metaphor for their passion, as they sway to the rhythm of their hearts, lost in the enchantment of each other's presence. Yet, like any great love story, their journey is not without challenges.

"Crossroads of Fate" tests their resolve, leading to moments of doubt and uncertainty. But through it all, their love prevails, stronger and more resilient than ever. In "Embracing the Unknown," they confront fears and insecurities, emerging victorious in their vulnerability.

Communication becomes key in "Lost in Translation," where misunderstandings pave the way for deeper understanding and empathy. And in "A Glimpse of Eternity," the timeless nature of their love is revealed—a love that transcends earthly constraints and touches the infinite.

Their paths intertwine in "Paths Intertwined," guided by the hand of destiny and the beauty of chance encounters. And in "Dreams Unfolding," they dare to dream of a future filled with endless possibilities, where love reigns supreme.

So, dear reader, buckle up and get ready for an unforgettable journey through "Unexpected Romance in Rio," where passion, resilience, and the magic of love await at every turn. The stage is set, the music plays on, and Carlos and Isabela's story is about to begin. Welcome to a world where love knows no limits and where every moment is an adventure waiting to unfold.

I

Carnival's Serendipity

The sun blazed overhead, casting a golden hue over the bustling streets of Rio de Janeiro. It was Carnival, the city's most anticipated event, where vibrant colors, infectious music, and joyful laughter filled every corner. Amidst the sea of revelers, two souls, unaware of each other's existence, were about to collide in a serendipitous twist of fate.

Carlos, a local musician with a passion for samba rhythms, was performing on a lively street corner. His fingers danced over the strings of his guitar, weaving melodies that echoed the pulsating energy of Carnival. His voice, rich and soulful, drew a crowd of admirers who swayed to the rhythm of his music.

Isabela, a free-spirited traveler from abroad, wandered through the crowded streets, her eyes wide with wonder at the spectacle unfolding around her. She had come to Rio seeking adventure, drawn by tales of Carnival's magic and the promise of unforgettable experiences.

As Isabela turned a corner, she stumbled upon Carlos's impromptu performance. Mesmerized by his talent and the infectious beat of his music, she found herself drawn closer, unable to tear her gaze away. Carlos, lost in the music and the euphoria of Carnival, glanced up and caught sight of Isabela's enraptured expression.

Their eyes met, and in that fleeting moment, a spark ignited between them. It was as if the universe conspired to bring two kindred spirits together in the midst of Carnival's chaos. Carlos felt a surge of inspiration, his music infused with newfound passion as he sang to Isabela, his lyrics weaving a tale of love and longing.

Isabela, captivated by Carlos's performance and the depth of emotion in his voice, felt her heartstrings resonate with the melody. She couldn't explain the magnetic pull she felt towards this stranger, but in that instant, she knew that Carnival had something extraordinary in store for her.

As the music faded into the background and the crowd cheered, Carlos and Isabela exchanged a shy smile, a silent acknowledgment of the connection that had sparked between them. Little did they know that this chance encounter was just the beginning of an unexpected romance that would unfold against the backdrop of Rio's pulsating energy.

Their story had begun, woven into the fabric of Carnival's exuberance, setting the stage for a journey filled with twists of fate, moments of serendipity, and the timeless magic of love found in unexpected places.

II

Echoes of the Night

As the sun dipped below the horizon, casting hues of orange and pink across the sky, the vibrant energy of Carnival transformed into a nocturnal symphony of lights and music. Carlos and Isabela's paths crossed once again, this time in the enchanting glow of Rio's nightlife.

Carlos had finished his performance for the day and decided to wander through the streets, his mind filled with the memory of Isabela's captivating presence. He couldn't shake off the feeling that their encounter was more than just a chance meeting—it was a sign from the universe.

Meanwhile, Isabela, still reeling from the magic of Carlos's music, roamed the streets with a sense of anticipation. She couldn't get the haunting melody out of her head, nor could she ignore the inexplicable pull she felt towards the mysterious musician.

As fate would have it, Carlos and Isabela found themselves in the same bustling square, surrounded by the pulsating rhythm of drums and the mesmerizing dance of revelers. Their eyes met once again, this time with a hint of recognition and curiosity.

Without a word, Carlos took Isabela's hand, leading her into the heart of the celebration. They danced under the starlit sky, their bodies moving in perfect harmony to the beat of the music. In that moment, time seemed to stand still as they lost themselves in the euphoria of the night.

Amidst the laughter and the joyous chaos of Carnival, Carlos and Isabela shared snippets of their lives—dreams, aspirations, and the hidden depths of their souls. Each word exchanged felt like a revelation, each glance a silent promise of something deeper yet to come.

As the night wore on, Carlos and Isabela found solace in each other's company, their connection growing stronger with every shared moment. They laughed, they danced, and they bared their vulnerabilities, creating a bond that transcended the fleeting nature of Carnival.

When the music finally faded and the crowds dispersed, Carlos and Isabela remained, reluctant to let go of the magic they had found in each other's arms. As they walked through the quiet streets, their footsteps echoing in the night, they knew that their unexpected romance was just beginning, a melody that would continue to play long after Carnival's echoes faded away.

III

Whispers of Doubt

In the days following Carnival, Carlos and Isabela found themselves navigating the delicate dance of uncertainty and anticipation. Their initial spark had ignited a flame of attraction and intrigue, but now they faced the challenge of turning that fleeting connection into something more tangible.

Carlos, haunted by the memory of Isabela's enchanting presence, struggled with doubts and insecurities. He wondered if their encounter during Carnival was simply a moment of fleeting magic, destined to fade into memory like so many other romances of the festival. Yet, deep down, he couldn't deny the longing in his heart for Isabela's laughter and the warmth of her gaze.

On the other hand, Isabela, caught in the whirlwind of her travels and adventures, found herself drawn back to Rio, to the memory of Carlos and the promise of something real amidst the transient beauty of Carnival. She replayed their moments together in her mind, searching for signs of a deeper connection beyond the enchantment of the festival.

Their paths crossed once again in a quiet café, where the melody of a guitar played softly in the background. Carlos, lost in thought, strummed the chords of a familiar tune, his eyes reflecting the tumult of emotions within. Isabela, drawn by the haunting melody, approached him with a hesitant smile.

Their conversation began tentatively, filled with unspoken questions and the weight of unspoken desires. Carlos shared snippets of his life—the passion for music that fueled his soul, the dreams he harbored, and the scars of past heartaches that made him cautious.

Isabela, in turn, opened up about her nomadic lifestyle, the thrill of exploration that fueled her wanderlust, and the longing for a connection that transcended borders and fleeting moments. Their words wove a tapestry of shared experiences, fears, and hopes for something more.

As the afternoon sun filtered through the café's windows, casting a warm glow over their table, Carlos and Isabela found solace in each other's company once again. Despite the whispers of doubt that lingered in the air, there was an undeniable chemistry between them—a connection that refused to be ignored.

They parted ways with a lingering promise—a tentative agreement to explore what lay between them, to see if their unexpected romance could withstand the tests of time and distance. As they walked away, their steps lighter with newfound hope, they knew that the journey ahead would be filled with challenges and uncertainties, but also the possibility of a love that defied expectations.

IV

Unveiling Vulnerabilities

In the days that followed their café encounter, Carlos and Isabela navigated the delicate balance between anticipation and hesitation. Each moment spent together revealed layers of vulnerability and strength, forging a bond that defied the transient nature of their initial meeting.

Carlos, determined to explore the depths of his connection with Isabela, invited her to a secluded spot overlooking the city. As they sat beneath the starlit sky, the city lights painting a mesmerizing backdrop, they delved into conversations that laid bare their innermost thoughts and emotions.

Isabela, usually so adventurous and free-spirited, found herself opening up in ways she hadn't anticipated. She shared stories of her past, the moments of joy and heartache that shaped her journey, and the longing for a love that felt like home amidst her nomadic lifestyle.

Carlos listened, his heart swelling with empathy and understanding. He, too, revealed parts of himself that he had kept guarded—the wounds of past relationships, the fear of vulnerability, and the hope that Isabela might be the one to break down his walls.

Their connection deepened with each shared confession, each moment of raw honesty weaving a stronger thread between them. They laughed together, cried together, and discovered the comfort of being truly seen and accepted for who they were, flaws and all.

As the night wore on, they moved from conversation to shared silences, their unspoken words carrying more weight than any spoken vow. In those quiet moments, Carlos and Isabela found solace in the simplicity of being together, their connection transcending the need for grand gestures or declarations.

When the first light of dawn painted the sky in hues of pink and gold, Carlos and Isabela sat in companionable silence, their hands intertwined, their hearts beating in sync. They knew that their journey was far from over, that challenges and obstacles lay ahead, but in that moment, all that mattered was the warmth of each other's presence.

As they watched the city awaken below them, Carlos and Isabela made a silent promise to cherish this unexpected romance, to nurture it with patience and understanding, and to let their love unfold organically, guided by the whispers of their hearts.

V

Embracing Challenges

As Carlos and Isabela's love story unfolded, they faced the inevitable challenges that tested the strength of their bond. With each obstacle, their connection deepened, revealing the resilience and depth of their feelings for each other.

One such challenge came in the form of distance. Isabela's nomadic lifestyle took her to distant lands, while Carlos remained rooted in Rio, pursuing his passion for music and navigating the complexities of their budding relationship.

Despite the miles that separated them, Carlos and Isabela stayed connected through letters, messages, and occasional video calls. Their communication became a lifeline, bridging the physical distance and keeping their love alive across continents.

In one heartfelt letter, Carlos poured out his emotions, expressing how much he missed Isabela's laughter, her presence, and the way she made his world brighter. Isabela, in turn, shared her adventures, the people she met, and the moments when she longed for nothing more than to be by Carlos's side.

Their love grew stronger with each passing day, fueled by the challenges they faced together and the unwavering commitment to make it work despite the odds. They learned to treasure every moment, whether it was a shared sunrise over video call or a handwritten letter that carried the scent of distant lands.

Yet, amidst the love and longing, doubts crept in. Would their love withstand the test of time and distance? Were they meant to be together despite the obstacles that stood in their way?

These questions lingered in their minds, adding a layer of complexity to their relationship. But through honest conversations and mutual reassurance, Carlos and Isabela found the strength to confront their doubts and reaffirm their commitment to each other.

In a poignant moment, Carlos surprised Isabela by flying to her current location, a gesture that spoke volumes of his love and dedication. Their reunion was filled with tears of joy, laughter, and the realization that no distance could diminish the depth of their connection.

As they embraced in each other's arms, surrounded by unfamiliar sights and sounds, Carlos and Isabela knew that their love was resilient, capable of weathering any storm. They had faced challenges head-on and emerged stronger, ready to continue their journey together, hand in hand, no matter where life took them.

VI

Navigating Crossroads

As Carlos and Isabela's love story unfolded across continents, they found themselves at a crossroads, facing decisions that would shape the course of their relationship and their individual journeys.

Isabela's travels had taken her to new and exciting places, each experience enriching her soul and fueling her sense of adventure. Yet, with every adventure came a longing for stability, for a place to call home and a person to share it with.

Carlos, too, grappled with conflicting emotions. His love for Isabela was unwavering, but he wondered if their different paths would eventually lead them in opposite directions. He longed for a future where they could build a life together, but the uncertainty of distance and time weighed heavily on his heart.

In a moment of vulnerability, Isabela shared her fears and dreams with Carlos, laying bare her desire for a life that balanced adventure and stability, freedom and commitment. Carlos listened with empathy, his own heart echoing her sentiments and yearning for a resolution.

Their conversations became more introspective, delving into their hopes, fears, and aspirations for the future. They explored possibilities, discussed compromises, and faced the reality that love sometimes requires sacrifice and courage.

One evening, as they watched the sunset together over a video call, Carlos made a heartfelt confession. He expressed his love for Isabela, his desire to build a future together, and his willingness to take the necessary steps to make it happen.

Isabela, deeply moved by Carlos's sincerity and love, made a decision of her own. She realized that home wasn't just a place—it was wherever her heart felt at peace, and that place was by Carlos's side.

With renewed determination and a shared vision for their future, Carlos and Isabela embarked on a journey of planning and preparation. They navigated visa applications, travel arrangements, and the logistics of merging their lives together, all while savoring the anticipation of a life filled with love, adventure, and companionship.

As they took each step forward, hand in hand, Carlos and Isabela knew that their love had withstood every challenge thrown their way. They had grown individually and as a couple, learning the true meaning of commitment, resilience, and the enduring power of love found in unexpected places.

Their journey was far from over, but with each chapter they wrote together, Carlos and Isabela knew that they were creating a love story that would stand the test of time, a testament to the magic of unexpected romance and the courage to follow their hearts.

VII

Embracing New Beginnings

With their plans for a shared future taking shape, Carlos and Isabela embarked on a new chapter of their love story—one filled with excitement, anticipation, and the promise of new beginnings.

As Isabela prepared to make the journey to Rio to be with Carlos, she felt a mix of emotions—joy at the prospect of finally being reunited, apprehension about the changes ahead, and a deep sense of gratitude for the love that had brought them together.

Carlos, too, eagerly awaited Isabela's arrival, his heart racing with anticipation as he imagined their life together in Rio. He prepared their home, filling it with touches that reflected their shared dreams and aspirations, creating a space where their love could blossom and thrive.

When Isabela finally arrived, their reunion was filled with tears of joy, laughter, and the overwhelming realization that their love had overcome every obstacle in its path. They embraced with a renewed sense of purpose, grateful for the journey that had led them to this moment.

Together, they explored Rio's vibrant streets, revisiting the places where their love story had begun—the café where they had shared intimate conversations, the square where they had danced under the stars, and the secluded spot overlooking the city where they had bared their souls to each other.

As they settled into their life together, Carlos and Isabela discovered the joys of everyday moments—the comfort of morning coffee shared on their balcony, the laughter that filled their home, and the quiet moments of intimacy that deepened their connection.

They navigated the challenges of merging their lives, learning to compromise, communicate, and grow together as a couple. Each day brought new discoveries, new adventures, and a deeper appreciation for the love that anchored them through it all.

Through it all, Carlos and Isabela's love story continued to evolve, their bond strengthening with each passing day. They faced challenges with resilience, celebrated victories with joy, and embraced every moment as a precious gift.

As they looked towards the future, hand in hand, Carlos and Isabela knew that their unexpected romance had blossomed into a love that was as enduring as it was extraordinary. Their journey was a testament to the power of love, the beauty of second chances, and the magic of finding home in each other's arms.

VIII

A Promise for Tomorrow

As Carlos and Isabela settled into their life together in Rio, their love story continued to unfold with a sense of deep fulfillment and joy. Each day brought new experiences, new challenges, and a reaffirmation of the bond that had brought them together.

Their shared home became a sanctuary—a place filled with laughter, love, and the echoes of their journey from chance encounter to enduring partnership. They decorated it with mementos of their travels, photographs capturing their happiest moments, and little reminders of the love that had transformed their lives.

Carlos, ever the romantic, surprised Isabela with gestures of love—a handwritten letter tucked into her favorite book, a spontaneous picnic by the beach at sunset, and impromptu serenades that echoed through their neighborhood, filling the air with music and passion.

Isabela, in turn, showered Carlos with her affection—a home-cooked meal that reminded him of his favorite childhood dish, a day of exploring hidden gems of Rio that she had discovered during her travels, and heartfelt conversations that deepened their connection even further.

Their love was a dance—a delicate balance of passion and tenderness, laughter and tears, shared dreams and individual aspirations. They supported each other's ambitions, celebrated each other's successes, and weathered life's challenges as a team, knowing that together, they were stronger.

As they reflected on their journey—the chance encounter at Carnival, the whirlwind of emotions and uncertainties, the challenges they had overcome, and the love that had blossomed against all odds—Carlos and Isabela knew that their love was a once-in-a-lifetime gift.

They made promises for tomorrow—a future filled with adventure, laughter, and unwavering devotion. They dreamed of traveling the world together, exploring new cultures, and creating memories that would last a lifetime.

But amidst their dreams, they cherished the present moment—the simple joys of everyday life, the warmth of each other's presence, and the knowledge that they had found their home in each other's hearts.

As they stood on their balcony, overlooking the vibrant city of Rio, Carlos and Isabela shared a quiet moment of gratitude—for the journey that had led them to each other, for the love that had blossomed and flourished, and for the promise of a tomorrow filled with endless possibilities.

Their love story was a testament to the power of love—unpredictable, transformative, and enduring. And as they looked towards the horizon, hand in hand, Carlos and Isabela knew that their love would continue to grow, evolve, and inspire, creating a legacy of love that would last a lifetime.

IX

A Celebration of Love

As Carlos and Isabela's love story continued to unfold, they found themselves at a moment of celebration—a time to reflect on their journey, honor their love, and embrace the future with open hearts.

Their shared home in Rio had become a sanctuary of love, filled with memories, laughter, and the echoes of their shared dreams. They often spent evenings reminiscing about their adventures, flipping through photo albums that captured their happiest moments together.

One evening, as they sat on their balcony, watching the city lights twinkle below, Carlos surprised Isabela with a special gift—a handmade journal filled with their love story. Each page was adorned with their favorite quotes, photographs, and handwritten notes that chronicled their journey from strangers to soulmates.

Isabela was moved to tears by Carlos's thoughtful gesture, touched by the effort he had put into capturing their love in such a beautiful way. They spent hours reading through the journal, reliving their most cherished memories and marveling at how far they had come.

Their love had weathered storms, faced challenges, and emerged stronger than ever. They had learned to communicate openly, to support each other's dreams, and to find joy in the simple moments of togetherness.

As they danced under the moonlit sky, their hearts overflowing with love and gratitude, Carlos whispered words of love and commitment to Isabela. He promised to always stand by her side, to cherish and protect their love, and to never take their relationship for granted.

Isabela, equally moved by Carlos's words, made her own vows of love and devotion. She promised to be his rock, his partner in adventure, and his source of unwavering support through life's ups and downs.

Their dance was a celebration of love—a dance of two souls entwined in a timeless rhythm, united by a bond that transcended words. They reveled in the magic of the moment, knowing that their love was a gift to be treasured for eternity.

As they embraced, the city of Rio shimmering in the background, Carlos and Isabela knew that their love story was far from over. It was a story of resilience, of growth, and of the endless possibilities that love could bring.

With hearts full of love and hope, Carlos and Isabela looked towards the future, ready to write new chapters of their love story, one filled with laughter, adventure, and the enduring power of love.

X

A Journey of Renewal

As Carlos and Isabela's love story continued to unfold, they embarked on a journey of renewal—a time of reflection, growth, and deepening their bond in ways they never imagined.

Their life together in Rio had become a tapestry of shared experiences, laughter, and the comfort of knowing they had found their forever in each other's arms. Yet, amidst the joy, they faced moments of introspection and growth that strengthened their love even further.

One day, as they explored a secluded beach outside of Rio, Carlos and Isabela found themselves immersed in the natural beauty that surrounded them. The crashing waves, the gentle breeze, and the vast expanse of the ocean mirrored the depth of their love and the endless possibilities that lay ahead.

As they walked hand in hand along the shore, Carlos and Isabela engaged in heartfelt conversations about their hopes, dreams, and the lessons they had learned along their journey. They talked about the importance of communication, trust, and the courage to face challenges together as a team.

Isabela shared her newfound sense of purpose—a desire to create meaningful impact through her travels, to give back to the communities she visited, and to inspire others to follow their passions with courage and compassion.

Carlos, inspired by Isabela's vision and resilience, opened up about his own dreams of using music as a tool for healing and connection.

He spoke of creating music that spoke to the soul, that transcended boundaries and brought people together in harmony.

Their conversations led to moments of introspection and renewal, as they reflected on their individual journeys and how they had grown together as a couple. They acknowledged the challenges they had faced, the moments of doubt and uncertainty, and the strength they had found in each other's love.

As the sun dipped below the horizon, casting a golden glow over the ocean, Carlos and Isabela made a pact—a promise to continue growing, learning, and evolving together. They vowed to support each other's dreams, to celebrate each other's successes, and to navigate life's twists and turns with grace and resilience.

Their journey of renewal was a testament to the transformative power of love—a love that had brought them together, guided them through challenges, and renewed their spirits with hope and determination.

As they stood on the beach, watching the stars twinkle above, Carlos and Isabela felt a renewed sense of purpose and passion for the future. Their love story was a journey of renewal—a journey that would continue to unfold, bringing them closer with each new chapter.

XI

Embracing Challenges Together

As Carlos and Isabela's love story evolved, they faced new challenges that tested their resilience and strengthened their bond. Each obstacle they encountered became an opportunity to grow closer, to learn more about themselves and each other, and to reaffirm their commitment to their relationship.

One such challenge came in the form of a career opportunity for Isabela that required her to travel extensively. While excited about the prospect of new experiences, Isabela also grappled with the idea of being away from Carlos for extended periods.

Carlos, understanding Isabela's passion for exploration and growth, encouraged her to pursue the opportunity wholeheartedly. He reassured her that their love was strong enough to withstand the distance, that they would find ways to stay connected despite the miles between them.

As Isabela embarked on her journey, Carlos made a conscious effort to support her from afar. They scheduled regular video calls, sent each other heartfelt messages and surprises, and found ways to keep the spark alive despite the challenges of distance.

Their love became a beacon of strength, guiding them through moments of doubt and loneliness. They learned to appreciate the value of quality time together, to cherish the moments they shared, and to communicate openly and honestly about their feelings.

As Isabela navigated her career path and Carlos continued to pursue his musical dreams in Rio, they found solace in the knowledge that their love was constant, unwavering, and filled with endless possibilities.

Their journey together became a testament to the power of love in overcoming obstacles, in embracing challenges as opportunities for growth, and in finding strength in each other's presence, no matter the distance.

As they looked towards the future, Carlos and Isabela knew that their love story was far from over. It was a story of resilience, of unwavering support, and of the enduring bond that held them together through life's highs and lows.

Their love was a testament to the fact that no challenge was too great, no distance too far, as long as they faced them together, hand in hand, with hearts full of love and determination.

XII

Finding Harmony in Differences

As Carlos and Isabela continued their journey together, they encountered moments where their differences brought them closer, enriching their relationship with new perspectives, experiences, and a deeper understanding of each other.

One of the areas where they found harmony in differences was their approach to creativity. Carlos, deeply immersed in the world of music, found inspiration in melodies, rhythms, and the emotions they evoked. Isabela, on the other hand, drew her creativity from the vastness of nature, the diversity of cultures she encountered in her travels, and the stories of people she met along the way.

Their differing creative processes initially posed challenges, as they struggled to find common ground in expressing their individual passions. However, they soon realized that their differences were not obstacles but opportunities to learn from each other, to grow together, and to create something truly unique.

Carlos began to incorporate Isabela's love for nature and cultural diversity into his music, infusing his melodies with global rhythms, exotic instruments, and themes that celebrated the beauty of the world they explored together. Isabela, in turn, found inspiration in Carlos's passion for music, weaving his melodies into her stories, capturing the emotions they stirred, and creating art that resonated with the heart.

Their collaboration became a harmonious dance of creativity, where each contributed their strengths, learned from each other's perspectives, and celebrated the beauty of their differences. They discovered that their love was not just about shared interests but about embracing and appreciating the unique qualities that made them who they were.

As they created together, Carlos and Isabela found a deeper connection, a shared language of creativity that transcended words, and a sense of fulfillment in knowing that their love was reflected in every note, every brushstroke, and every word they shared.

Their journey of finding harmony in differences became a metaphor for their relationship—a beautiful tapestry woven from threads of love, understanding, and the willingness to embrace each other's differences as strengths.

As they looked back on their journey, from the chance encounter at Carnival to the moments of growth, challenges, and love that had shaped their story, Carlos and Isabela knew that their love was a masterpiece in the making—a work of art that would continue to evolve, inspire, and resonate with the world.

XIII
Navigating Life's Crossroads

As Carlos and Isabela's love story continued to unfold, they found themselves at a crossroads once again—a moment of reflection, decision, and the realization that their journey together was filled with twists, turns, and unexpected blessings.

One of the challenges they faced was balancing their individual dreams with their shared life. Carlos's music career was thriving, with opportunities to perform in prestigious venues and collaborate with renowned artists. Isabela's passion for travel and exploration led her to new adventures and opportunities to make a difference in the world.

Their busy schedules sometimes created moments of longing and separation, as they navigated the demands of their respective passions. Yet, they also found strength in their shared commitment to supporting each other's dreams, to finding a balance that honored their individual paths while nurturing their relationship.

Carlos and Isabela had honest conversations about their goals, aspirations, and the compromises they were willing to make for each other. They acknowledged the challenges of pursuing their dreams while maintaining a strong connection, but they also recognized that their love was a source of inspiration, motivation, and unwavering support.

Together, they navigated life's crossroads with grace and determination, finding creative ways to stay connected despite the distance and time apart. They sent each other messages of love and encouragement, surprised each other with thoughtful gestures, and made plans for moments of togetherness amidst their busy schedules.

Their love became a beacon of stability, guiding them through moments of uncertainty and doubt. They learned to appreciate the value of quality time, to cherish the moments they shared, and to trust in the strength of their bond no matter where life took them.

As they stood at the crossroads of their journey, Carlos and Isabela made a vow to continue supporting each other, to celebrate their individual successes as well as their shared victories, and to navigate life's challenges with resilience, love, and a deep sense of gratitude for the journey they had embarked on together.

Their love story was not just about romance—it was about growth, partnership, and the courage to follow their dreams while holding onto each other's hands through it all.

XIV

Laughter in the Rain

Amidst the challenges and decisions they faced, Carlos and Isabela also found moments of laughter, joy, and unexpected humor that added color to their journey.

One rainy evening in Rio, as they were caught in a sudden downpour without an umbrella, Carlos and Isabela found themselves drenched but laughing uncontrollably. They sought refuge under a nearby awning, their laughter echoing through the empty streets as they embraced the absurdity of the situation.

Isabela's infectious laughter, coupled with Carlos's playful jokes, turned what could have been a dreary moment into a memory they would cherish forever. They danced in the rain, sang silly songs, and made a promise to always find humor in life's unexpected twists and turns.

Their laughter became a symbol of resilience, a reminder that even in the midst of challenges, there was always room for joy and lightheartedness. They embraced each other with warmth and affection, their spirits lifted by the simple act of sharing laughter in the rain.

As they walked home, hand in hand, their clothes clinging to their bodies, Carlos and Isabela knew that their love was not just about weathering storms but about finding moments of happiness and laughter even in the darkest of times.

XV

Echoes of Melancholy

Despite the moments of laughter and joy, Carlos and Isabela also experienced periods of sadness and melancholy, reminding them of the depth of their emotions and the complexities of life.

One evening, as they sat by the window watching the rain cascade down, a wave of nostalgia washed over them. They found themselves reminiscing about the past—memories of loved ones no longer with them, moments of missed opportunities, and the bittersweet ache of longing for what could have been.

Isabela's eyes glistened with unshed tears as she spoke of her late grandmother, a woman whose love and wisdom had shaped her in profound ways. Carlos held her hand, his own heart heavy with memories of his father, whose absence was felt acutely in quiet moments like these.

Together, they allowed themselves to feel the weight of their emotions, to acknowledge the sadness that lingered in their hearts, and to find solace in each other's presence. They shared stories, whispered words of comfort, and found strength in the knowledge that their love could weather even the stormiest of emotions.

Their sadness became a reminder of the depth of their love—a love that embraced both the light and the shadows, the laughter and the tears. They held onto each other with renewed tenderness, grateful for the moments of vulnerability that deepened their connection.

As the rain continued to fall outside, Carlos and Isabela found solace in music. They played songs that spoke to their hearts, that echoed their emotions, and that served as a cathartic release for the sadness they carried.

In those moments of shared sorrow, Carlos and Isabela discovered a profound truth—that love was not just about happiness and laughter but about being there for each other in times of sadness, offering comfort, understanding, and a shoulder to lean on.

As they curled up together, the rain tapping gently on the window, Carlos and Isabela felt a sense of peace wash over them. Their love had weathered another storm, proving once again that even in sadness, there was beauty, connection, and the enduring strength of their bond.

XVI

The Dance of Renewal

After moments of laughter and tears, Carlos and Isabela found themselves embracing a period of renewal—a time to rediscover themselves, their love, and the endless possibilities that lay ahead.

They embarked on a journey of self-discovery, exploring new interests, hobbies, and passions that added richness and depth to their relationship. Carlos delved deeper into his music, experimenting with new sounds, collaborating with local artists, and finding inspiration in the vibrant energy of Rio's music scene.

Isabela, too, pursued her love for storytelling, capturing the essence of their love story in a series of paintings that reflected their journey—from the colorful chaos of Carnival to the quiet moments of introspection and connection.

Their individual pursuits brought them closer, as they supported each other's creative endeavors, celebrated each other's successes, and found new ways to inspire and uplift one another.

One evening, as they attended a local dance performance, Carlos and Isabela were captivated by the graceful movements, the passion in the music, and the storytelling through dance. Inspired by the performance, they decided to take dance lessons together, immersing themselves in the joy of movement, rhythm, and the intimate connection that dance fostered between them.

Their dance became a metaphor for their relationship—a beautiful blend of harmony, passion, and the joy of being in sync with each other's hearts. They twirled, dipped, and embraced on the dance floor, lost in the moment and the music that spoke to their souls.

Through dance, Carlos and Isabela discovered new layers of intimacy, trust, and communication. They learned to express their emotions without words, to move in unison, and to find joy in the simple act of being together, moving as one.

As they danced under the starlit sky, Carlos and Isabela felt a sense of renewal wash over them—a renewal of their love, their connection, and their shared vision for the future. They knew that their journey was far from over, but they also knew that as long as they danced through life together, they would always find renewal, growth, and the magic of unexpected romance in Rio.

XVII

Whispers of Tomorrow

As Carlos and Isabela continued their journey of renewal and growth, they found themselves drawn to the whispers of tomorrow—a sense of anticipation, excitement, and the promise of new beginnings.

One afternoon, as they strolled through a botanical garden in Rio, surrounded by lush greenery and blooming flowers, they talked about their dreams for the future. They shared visions of traveling the world together, exploring new cultures, and creating a life filled with adventure, love, and endless possibilities.

Their conversations were filled with excitement and enthusiasm, as they mapped out their dreams, set goals, and made plans for the adventures that awaited them. They talked about the places they wanted to visit, the experiences they wanted to have, and the memories they wanted to create together.

Isabela expressed her desire to use her storytelling and artistic talents to inspire others, to create art that touched hearts and minds, and to make a positive impact on the world. Carlos shared his vision of using music as a tool for healing, connection, and spreading joy to people from all walks of life.

Together, they made a pact to support each other's dreams wholeheartedly, to be each other's biggest cheerleaders, and to never lose sight of the magic they had found in each other's arms.

As they sat on a bench overlooking a serene pond, the sun setting in the distance, Carlos and Isabela felt a sense of peace and contentment wash over them. They knew that the road ahead would have its challenges, its ups and downs, but they also knew that as long as they faced them together, hand in hand, they could conquer anything.

Their whispers of tomorrow became a promise—a promise to live life to the fullest, to embrace new adventures with open hearts, and to cherish every moment they shared together.

As they left the botanical garden, their hearts filled with hope and excitement for the future, Carlos and Isabela knew that their love story was far from over. It was a story of resilience, growth, and the enduring power of love to light the way to tomorrow's dreams.

XVIII

Serendipity's Embrace

As Carlos and Isabela embarked on their journey towards tomorrow's dreams, they were met with serendipitous moments that reminded them of the beauty of life's unexpected twists and turns.

One sunny afternoon, while exploring a hidden gem of a bookstore in Rio, Carlos stumbled upon a rare vinyl record—one that held sentimental value from his childhood. The discovery brought a smile to his face, a rush of nostalgia, and a deep sense of connection to his past and present.

Isabela, sensing the significance of the find, joined Carlos in marveling at the record's artwork, its vintage charm, and the memories it evoked. Together, they decided to purchase the record as a symbol of their journey—a reminder that life often brought treasures in the most unexpected places.

As they left the bookstore, Carlos and Isabela found themselves caught in a spontaneous dance on the bustling streets of Rio. Their laughter echoed through the crowds, their feet moving in sync to the rhythm of the city, and their hearts filled with a sense of joy and gratitude for the serendipity that had brought them together.

Their dance became a celebration of life's surprises, of the small moments that brought immense happiness, and of the beauty of being open to the unexpected. They twirled, laughed, and embraced, their love shining brightly for all to see.

In that moment of serendipity's embrace, Carlos and Isabela realized that their love story was a testament to the magic of chance, the power of connection, and the joy of living life to the fullest.

As they watched the sunset paint the sky in hues of orange and pink, Carlos and Isabela knew that every twist and turn, every moment of laughter and tears, had led them to this beautiful chapter in their love story—a chapter filled with serendipitous moments and the promise of more adventures to come.

XIX

Embracing the Unknown

As Carlos and Isabela embraced the serendipitous moments that colored their journey, they also found themselves facing the unknown—a realm of possibilities, challenges, and the thrill of stepping into uncharted territory together.

One evening, as they sat on their balcony overlooking the city lights of Rio, Carlos and Isabela talked about their dreams for the future. They shared their hopes of traveling to new destinations, experiencing different cultures, and immersing themselves in the richness of life's adventures.

Yet, amidst the excitement of the unknown, there lingered a sense of apprehension—an acknowledgment of the uncertainties that lay ahead, the fears of the unfamiliar, and the courage it would take to navigate the uncharted waters of their dreams.

Isabela spoke of her desire to explore remote places, to venture off the beaten path, and to discover hidden gems that spoke to the soul. Carlos, too, expressed his yearning for new musical horizons, for collaborations that pushed boundaries, and for experiences that challenged and inspired him.

Together, they made a pact to embrace the unknown with open hearts, to see each challenge as an opportunity for growth, and to support each other's aspirations with unwavering faith and determination.

Their conversation turned to moments of humor as they recounted past adventures, shared funny anecdotes, and laughed at the quirks and idiosyncrasies that made them who they were. In the midst of uncertainty, their laughter became a source of strength, a reminder that no matter what life threw their way, they could face it together with joy and resilience.

As they gazed at the starry sky above, Carlos and Isabela felt a sense of anticipation mingled with excitement. The unknown was no longer a source of fear but a canvas waiting to be painted with the colors of their dreams, their love guiding them through every twist and turn.

Their embrace of the unknown was a testament to their courage, their faith in each other, and the belief that together, they could conquer anything that lay on the horizon of their shared journey.

XX

A Tapestry of Memories

As Carlos and Isabela ventured into the unknown, they found themselves weaving a tapestry of memories—a collection of moments, experiences, and emotions that formed the fabric of their love story.

Their journey took them to new places, each one leaving an indelible mark on their hearts. From the bustling streets of Rio to the serene beauty of remote villages, Carlos and Isabela embraced every adventure with open arms and open hearts.

One day, while exploring a quaint town nestled in the mountains, they stumbled upon a hidden café with a view that took their breath away. They sat at a table overlooking a panoramic vista of valleys and rivers, the sun painting the sky in hues of gold and amber.

As they sipped their coffee and savored the moment, Carlos and Isabela reflected on the memories they had created together—the laughter, the tears, the challenges, and the triumphs. They spoke of their love story as a journey of growth, resilience, and the deepening of their bond with each passing day.

Isabela captured the beauty of the scene in her paintings, each stroke of her brush imbued with the emotions they felt in that moment. Carlos composed a melody inspired by the tranquility of the mountains, the melody weaving through the air like a gentle breeze.

Their art became a reflection of their love, a testament to the richness of their experiences, and a treasure trove of memories to cherish for a lifetime. They knew that no matter where life took them, they would always have these moments to look back on and smile.

As they returned to Rio, their hearts full of gratitude for the memories they had created, Carlos and Isabela felt a deep sense of fulfillment. Their love story was not just about the destination but about the journey—the journey of discovery, growth, and the beauty of sharing life's moments together.

Their tapestry of memories was a testament to the depth of their love, the richness of their experiences, and the endless possibilities that lay ahead as they continued to write the chapters of their love story.

XXI

The Rhythm of Love

As Carlos and Isabela reflected on their tapestry of memories, they found themselves attuned to the rhythm of love—a melody that wove through their lives, connecting past, present, and future in harmonious resonance.

Their days were filled with music, laughter, and moments of quiet contemplation. Carlos's music filled their home with melodies that spoke of love, hope, and the beauty of shared dreams. Isabela's paintings adorned their walls, each canvas a window into their journey, their emotions, and their unwavering connection.

One evening, as they sat on their balcony under a starlit sky, Carlos picked up his guitar and began to play a new composition—a song that captured the essence of their love, the ups and downs, the joys and sorrows, and the unwavering bond that held them together.

Isabela listened, her heart swelling with love and gratitude for the man who had become her partner, her confidant, and her soulmate. She felt the music wash over her like a gentle breeze, carrying with it the memories of their journey and the promise of tomorrow's dreams.

Their dance of love continued, each step a testament to their commitment, their resilience, and their ability to find beauty in every note, every brushstroke, and every shared moment.

As they danced on their balcony, the city lights below twinkling in the distance, Carlos and Isabela felt a sense of peace and contentment wash over them. They knew that their love story was far from over, that new chapters awaited them, and that as long as they danced to the rhythm of love, they would always find joy, passion, and the magic of unexpected romance in Rio.

Their love was a symphony—an ever-evolving masterpiece that resonated with the melody of their hearts, the harmony of their souls, and the timeless beauty of love in all its forms.

XXII

Echoes of Tomorrow

As Carlos and Isabela embraced the rhythm of love, they were surrounded by echoes of tomorrow—a symphony of possibilities, dreams, and the endless horizon of their shared future.

Their days were filled with moments of creativity, laughter, and quiet conversations that deepened their bond. Carlos continued to compose music that spoke of their journey, while Isabela's paintings evolved into intricate tapestries of emotions and memories.

One day, as they walked along the shores of Rio's beaches, they marveled at the beauty of the sunset painting the sky in vibrant hues. They talked about their dreams for tomorrow, the places they wanted to explore, and the adventures that awaited them.

Isabela expressed her desire to create an art exhibition showcasing their love story, a visual journey through the moments that had defined their relationship. Carlos shared his vision of composing a symphony inspired by their experiences, a musical ode to their love and the city that had brought them together.

Together, they made plans for the future—traveling to distant lands, collaborating on creative projects, and continuing to grow as individuals while nurturing their relationship.

Their conversation turned to moments of humor as they reminisced about past adventures, shared funny anecdotes, and laughed at the quirks that made them uniquely themselves. In their laughter, they found solace, connection, and the joy of being together on this journey called life.

As they watched the waves caress the shore, Carlos and Isabela felt a sense of anticipation for what tomorrow held. Their love story was a tapestry woven with threads of laughter, tears, dreams, and moments of pure joy.

Their echoes of tomorrow were a promise—a promise to embrace every moment, to cherish every memory, and to continue writing the chapters of their love story with passion, resilience, and unwavering devotion.

XXIII
Whispers of Destiny

As Carlos and Isabela stood on the threshold of tomorrow, they were enveloped by whispers of destiny—a gentle reminder of the paths they had walked, the choices they had made, and the unspoken promise of what lay ahead.

Their days were filled with a sense of purpose, as they delved deeper into their creative pursuits and shared dreams. Carlos's music filled their home with melodies that echoed their love story, while Isabela's art continued to capture the nuances of their journey.

One evening, as they sat under a canopy of stars in Rio's botanical garden, Carlos and Isabela spoke of destiny and the role it had played in bringing them together. They talked about the moments of serendipity, the chance encounters, and the threads of fate that had woven their lives into a beautiful tapestry.

Isabela expressed her belief in the interconnectedness of events, the way each choice led to another, and the magic of following one's heart. Carlos nodded in agreement, sharing his belief that destiny was not just about preordained paths but about the choices they made along the way, the courage to take risks, and the willingness to embrace the unknown.

Their conversation turned to moments of reflection as they looked back on their journey—the highs and lows, the laughter and tears, and the unwavering love that had sustained them through it all. In each memory, they found a thread of destiny, a guiding light that had led them to where they were now.

As they walked hand in hand through the garden, surrounded by the fragrance of flowers and the whisper of leaves, Carlos and Isabela felt a sense of gratitude for the journey they had shared. Their love story was not just a series of moments but a testament to the power of destiny, the beauty of connection, and the strength of their bond.

Their whispers of destiny were a reminder that their paths had crossed for a reason, that their love was written in the stars, and that together, they could conquer anything that destiny had in store for them.

XXIV

Embracing the Stars

As Carlos and Isabela pondered destiny's whispers, they found themselves drawn to the celestial beauty above—a reminder of the vastness of the universe, the mysteries it held, and the interconnectedness of all things.

Their days became infused with a sense of wonder as they gazed at the stars, contemplating the stories they held and the secrets they whispered. Carlos's music took on celestial themes, his melodies echoing the dance of planets and the harmony of cosmic forces.

One night, as they lay on a blanket under the starry sky, Carlos pointed out constellations, sharing stories and myths from different cultures. Isabela listened, captivated by the tales of love, adventure, and the enduring presence of the stars throughout history.

They talked about their own journey, how their love had navigated through moments of light and darkness, how it had endured challenges and grown stronger with each passing day. Isabela spoke of the stars as symbols of hope, guiding lights in times of uncertainty, and reminders of the beauty that existed beyond earthly concerns.

Carlos nodded in agreement, his eyes reflecting the starlight as he expressed his belief in the interconnectedness of all things, the way the universe conspired to bring souls together, and the magic that existed in every moment shared with Isabela.

Their conversation turned to moments of laughter as they shared funny anecdotes about their adventures under the stars, the missteps and mishaps that had only served to deepen their connection and add to their shared memories.

As they lay side by side, the night alive with the symphony of crickets and the twinkling of stars, Carlos and Isabela felt a profound sense of unity with the cosmos. Their love story was a reflection of the stars—eternal, radiant, and filled with the promise of endless possibilities.

Their embrace of the stars was a testament to their belief in something greater than themselves, in the beauty of the unknown, and in the enduring power of love to illuminate even the darkest of nights.

XXV

Whispers of Eternity

As Carlos and Isabela embraced the celestial wonders above, they felt whispers of eternity caress their souls—a reminder of the timeless nature of love, the enduring connection they shared, and the depth of their bond that transcended the boundaries of time.

Their days were filled with moments of quiet contemplation, as they explored the deeper meanings of their love and the mysteries of the universe. Carlos's music took on a soulful quality, his melodies reflecting the depth of emotion and the longing for a love that spanned lifetimes.

One evening, as they sat by a bonfire on the beach, the waves crashing gently in the background, Carlos and Isabela spoke of eternity and the infinite possibilities it held. They talked about the concept of soulmates, of souls destined to find each other across time and space, and of the profound connection they felt in each other's presence.

Isabela expressed her belief in the continuity of love, the idea that even beyond this lifetime, their souls would find each other again and again. Carlos nodded in agreement, his eyes reflecting the flames of the fire as he spoke of the timeless nature of their bond, the way their love had endured through trials and tribulations, and the certainty that it would continue to flourish for eternity.

Their conversation turned to moments of reflection as they shared memories from past lives—dreams that felt like memories, inexplicable connections, and the sense of déjà vu that had accompanied their meeting in this lifetime. In each memory, they found echoes of their love, whispers of eternity that bound them together across the ages.

As they watched the stars above, the constellations shifting in a dance of cosmic beauty, Carlos and Isabela felt a sense of peace and completeness. Their love story was not just a chapter in time but a saga that stretched across eternity, a testament to the enduring power of love to transcend all boundaries.

Their whispers of eternity were a promise—a promise of love that knew no limits, of a connection that defied time, and of a bond that would continue to shine like a beacon through the ages.

XXVI

A Promise in the Sand

As Carlos and Isabela basked in the whispers of eternity, they found themselves drawn to the timeless beauty of nature—a canvas where their love story unfolded, leaving traces of promises in the sands of time.

Their days were filled with moments of tranquility, as they wandered along Rio's pristine beaches, their footsteps leaving imprints in the soft sand. Carlos's music echoed the rhythm of the waves, a melody that spoke of love's enduring strength and the passage of time.

One afternoon, as they walked hand in hand along the shore, Carlos stopped to draw a heart in the sand, inside of which he wrote "Carlos and Isabela, forever." Isabela smiled, her eyes shimmering with tears of joy as she added her own message next to his, "Together, always."

They stood there, watching the waves gently wash over their declaration, knowing that while the sands may shift and change, their love remained steadfast and unyielding.

Their conversation turned to moments of gratitude as they expressed their appreciation for each other, for the journey they had shared, and for the deep connection that bound them together. Isabela spoke of the strength she found in Carlos's love, the way he had been her rock through life's storms. Carlos, in turn, thanked Isabela for bringing light and joy into his world, for inspiring him to be the best version of himself.

Their words were a promise—a promise to stand by each other's side through thick and thin, to weather life's challenges together, and to cherish every moment as a gift.

As they walked back to their home, the sun setting in a blaze of colors, Carlos and Isabela felt a sense of peace and fulfillment. Their love story was not just about grand gestures but about the simple, heartfelt promises they made to each other every day.

Their promise in the sand was a symbol—a symbol of their commitment, their devotion, and the enduring power of love to leave its mark on the sands of time.

XXVII

Harmony of Hearts

As Carlos and Isabela cherished the promise they made in the sand, they found themselves immersed in the harmony of their hearts—a melody that echoed through every moment, every word, and every glance shared between them.

Their days were filled with a sense of contentment, as they embraced the beauty of everyday life and the comfort of being in each other's presence. Carlos's music took on a softer tone, a symphony of love that resonated with the rhythm of their hearts.

One evening, as they sat on their balcony overlooking Rio's city lights, Carlos picked up his guitar and began to play a familiar tune—a song that had become their anthem, a melody that spoke of love's enduring grace and the journey they had traveled together.

Isabela listened, her heart swelling with emotion as she looked at Carlos, their eyes meeting in a silent exchange of love and understanding. She knew in that moment that their bond was unbreakable, their connection woven into the very fabric of their souls.

Their conversation turned to moments of reflection as they talked about the challenges they had faced and the growth they had experienced as individuals and as a couple. Isabela spoke of the strength they had found in each other, the way their love had been a source of courage and resilience in times of adversity. Carlos, too, shared his gratitude for Isabela's unwavering support, her kindness, and the way she had brought light into his life.

Their words were a harmony—a harmony of hearts beating as one, of souls intertwined in a dance of love and devotion. In their togetherness, they found solace, joy, and the promise of a future filled with shared dreams and continued growth.

As they watched the stars twinkle above, a sense of peace washed over them. Their love story was a symphony—a symphony of laughter and tears, of challenges and triumphs, and above all, of love that knew no bounds.

Their harmony of hearts was a testament—a testament to the enduring power of love, the beauty of connection, and the magic of finding a soulmate who completes you in every way.

XXVIII

The Dance of Dreams

As Carlos and Isabela reveled in the harmony of their hearts, they found themselves swept up in the dance of dreams—a waltz of aspirations, hopes, and the shared vision of a future filled with love and possibilities.

Their days were imbued with a sense of anticipation, as they embarked on new adventures and pursued their passions with renewed fervor. Carlos's music took on a buoyant rhythm, a melody that echoed the joy of pursuing dreams alongside a beloved partner.

One sunny afternoon, as they strolled through Rio's bustling streets, Carlos and Isabela found themselves drawn to a dance studio, its doors open invitingly. Without hesitation, they stepped inside, eager to explore the world of dance together.

Under the guidance of a skilled instructor, Carlos and Isabela swayed to the music, their bodies moving in synchrony, their eyes locked in a dance of shared joy and connection. With each step, they felt a sense of unity, a blending of energies that spoke of their deep bond and mutual understanding.

Their conversation turned to moments of excitement as they talked about their dreams for the future—the places they wanted to visit, the projects they wanted to undertake, and the adventures that awaited them. Isabela expressed her desire to travel to distant lands, to immerse herself in different cultures, and to capture the beauty of the world through her art. Carlos shared his dream of composing music that transcended boundaries, that spoke to the hearts of people from all walks of life.

Their dreams became intertwined—a tapestry of shared aspirations, mutual support, and the belief that together, they could achieve anything they set their minds to.

As they twirled across the dance floor, the music guiding their movements, Carlos and Isabela felt a sense of exhilaration. Their love story was not just about the present but about the endless possibilities that lay ahead, the dreams they shared, and the joy of pursuing them together.

Their dance of dreams was a celebration—a celebration of love, of unity, and of the beauty that comes from embracing life's adventures hand in hand.

XXIX

Echoes of Laughter

As Carlos and Isabela continued their dance of dreams, they found themselves surrounded by echoes of laughter—a chorus of joy, playfulness, and the shared moments of light-heartedness that added color to their love story.

Their days were filled with laughter, as they discovered the humor in everyday situations and embraced the joy of being together. Carlos's music took on playful notes, a melody that mirrored the laughter that bubbled between them.

One evening, as they dined at a lively restaurant in Rio, Carlos and Isabela found themselves sharing stories and jokes, their laughter mingling with the cheerful ambiance of the place. They talked about funny moments from their past adventures, the mishaps and surprises that had brought them closer together, and the joy of finding humor even in challenging times.

Their conversation turned to moments of light-heartedness as they reminisced about their shared sense of humor, the inside jokes that only they understood, and the way laughter had become a constant companion in their relationship. Isabela expressed her gratitude for Carlos's ability to make her laugh, to lighten her mood even on the darkest days. Carlos, in turn, thanked Isabela for bringing joy and playfulness into his life, for reminding him to not take things too seriously.

Their laughter became a symphony—a symphony of shared joy, of playful banter, and of the deep connection that allowed them to be themselves completely.

As they walked along the bustling streets of Rio, their laughter ringing out like music, Carlos and Isabela felt a sense of unity and warmth. Their love story was not just about serious moments but about the laughter that added sparkle to their days, the jokes that created memories, and the joy of simply being together.

Their echoes of laughter were a reminder—a reminder to find joy in the little things, to laugh often, and to embrace the playful spirit that kept their love alive and vibrant.

XXX

Serenade of Serenity

As Carlos and Isabela reveled in the echoes of laughter, they found themselves enveloped in a serenade of serenity—a melody of peace, tranquility, and the deep sense of contentment that came from being with the one you love.

Their days took on a slower pace, as they embraced moments of quietude and reflection. Carlos's music transitioned into soothing tunes, a serenade that calmed their souls and spoke of the harmony they found in each other's presence.

One afternoon, as they lounged in their garden, surrounded by the fragrance of blooming flowers, Carlos picked up his guitar and began to play a gentle melody. Isabela closed her eyes, letting the music wash over her, feeling a sense of peace settle in her heart.

Their conversation turned to moments of serenity as they talked about the importance of finding quiet moments amidst life's busyness, of appreciating the beauty of nature, and of cherishing the stillness shared between them. Isabela expressed her gratitude for Carlos's calming presence, for the way he always knew how to soothe her worries and bring her back to a place of peace. Carlos, too, thanked Isabela for being his anchor, for grounding him in moments of chaos and reminding him of the beauty of simplicity.

Their words were a serenade—a serenade of gratitude, of love, and of the deep connection that allowed them to find solace in each other's arms.

As they watched the sun dip below the horizon, painting the sky in hues of orange and pink, Carlos and Isabela felt a profound sense of harmony. Their love story was not just about excitement and laughter but about the quiet moments shared, the moments of serenity that strengthened their bond and nourished their souls.

Their serenade of serenity was a gift—a gift of tranquility, of appreciation for each other, and of the profound love that blossomed in the stillness of their hearts.

XXXI

Embracing the Dance of Life

As Carlos and Isabela immersed themselves in the serenade of serenity, they found themselves embracing the dance of life—a graceful waltz of acceptance, growth, and the beauty of experiencing every moment together.

Their days became a canvas of experiences, as they embraced new challenges and celebrated small victories. Carlos's music evolved into a symphony of life's rhythms, a melody that mirrored the ever-changing nature of their journey.

One day, as they explored a local art gallery, Carlos and Isabela found themselves captivated by a painting that depicted a dance—figures twirling in perfect harmony, their movements fluid and synchronized. They stood in front of the painting, feeling a connection to the artist's portrayal of life as a dance, with its ups and downs, its moments of grace and unpredictability.

Their conversation turned to moments of reflection as they talked about the dance of life—the way it ebbed and flowed, the lessons it taught them, and the growth they experienced through its twists and turns. Isabela expressed her gratitude for the richness of their experiences, for the way each moment, whether joyful or challenging, contributed to their journey together. Carlos nodded in agreement, sharing his belief in the beauty of embracing life fully, of savoring every emotion and embracing every opportunity for growth.

Their words were a dance—a dance of acceptance, of resilience, and of the deep connection that allowed them to navigate life's complexities with grace and courage.

As they left the gallery, the sun casting a warm glow over the city, Carlos and Isabela felt a sense of unity with the world around them. Their love story was not just about their relationship but about their shared experience of life, the dance they embraced together, and the beauty of living in the present moment.

Their embrace of the dance of life was a celebration—a celebration of growth, of resilience, and of the profound love that guided them through every step of their journey.

XXXII

Harmony in Adversity

As Carlos and Isabela embraced the dance of life, they found themselves discovering harmony even in moments of adversity—a testament to the strength of their bond and the resilience of their love.

Their days were filled with challenges, as life presented them with unexpected twists and turns. Carlos's music took on a somber yet hopeful tone, a melody that mirrored their journey through difficult times.

One evening, as they faced a setback together, Carlos and Isabela sat down to talk, their hearts heavy yet determined. They spoke of the challenges they were facing, the doubts and fears that crept in, and the uncertainty of what lay ahead. But amidst it all, they found solace in each other's presence, in the unwavering support they offered each other.

Their conversation turned to moments of strength as they shared stories of overcoming obstacles in the past, of finding silver linings in difficult situations, and of the resilience that had always carried them through. Isabela expressed her gratitude for Carlos's unwavering support, for being her rock when she needed it most. Carlos, too, thanked Isabela for her strength and determination, for inspiring him to keep pushing forward even in the face of adversity.

Their words were a symphony—a symphony of resilience, of courage, and of the deep connection that allowed them to weather life's storms together.

As they sat in silence, the weight of their challenges lifting slightly, Carlos and Isabela felt a sense of unity and determination. Their love story was not just about happy moments but about facing challenges head-on, about finding strength in each other, and about growing stronger together.

Their harmony in adversity was a reminder—a reminder that even in life's darkest moments, love could be a beacon of hope, guiding them through the storm and into brighter days ahead.

XXXIII

The Healing Power of Love

As Carlos and Isabela navigated through the challenges of adversity, they discovered the healing power of love—a force that brought solace, comfort, and renewal to their hearts.

Their days were marked by moments of introspection and growth, as they sought to mend the wounds left by life's trials. Carlos's music took on a gentle, soothing melody, a reflection of the healing journey they embarked upon together.

One rainy afternoon, as they sat by the window watching the raindrops cascade down, Carlos and Isabela engaged in a heartfelt conversation about healing. They spoke of the scars they carried, both visible and invisible, and the process of finding healing through love, understanding, and acceptance.

Their conversation turned to moments of vulnerability as they shared their deepest fears, regrets, and hopes for the future. Isabela expressed her gratitude for Carlos's patience and kindness, for being a constant source of support and reassurance. Carlos, too, thanked Isabela for her resilience and for teaching him the importance of self-love and forgiveness.

Their words were a balm—a balm that soothed their souls, healed old wounds, and brought a sense of peace and acceptance into their lives.

As they sat in comfortable silence, the rain washing away the remnants of pain, Carlos and Isabela felt a profound sense of renewal.

Their love story was not just about overcoming challenges but about the transformative power of love to heal, to mend broken pieces, and to create a future filled with hope and joy.

Their healing power of love was a testament—a testament to the resilience of the human spirit, the capacity for growth and renewal, and the enduring strength of their bond.

XXXIV
Embracing New Beginnings

As Carlos and Isabela experienced the healing power of love, they found themselves embracing new beginnings—a journey of renewal, growth, and the excitement of what the future held for them.

Their days were filled with a sense of optimism and possibility, as they let go of past hurts and embraced the opportunities that lay ahead. Carlos's music took on a hopeful melody, a reflection of the newfound joy and anticipation in their hearts.

One sunny morning, as they walked through a park adorned with blooming flowers, Carlos and Isabela talked about their dreams for the future. They spoke of new adventures they wanted to embark upon, new experiences they wanted to savor, and the joy of starting afresh.

Their conversation turned to moments of gratitude as they expressed appreciation for the journey they had been on, for the lessons learned, and for the strength they had gained from facing challenges together. Isabela spoke of her excitement for the possibilities that lay ahead, for the chance to create new memories and write new chapters in their love story. Carlos, too, shared his enthusiasm for the future, for the chance to explore the world with Isabela by his side, and to build a life filled with love and purpose.

Their words were a beacon—a beacon of hope, of renewal, and of the endless possibilities that awaited them as they stepped into a new chapter of their lives.

As they sat on a bench, watching children play and laughter fill the air, Carlos and Isabela felt a sense of anticipation and joy. Their love story was not just about overcoming obstacles but about embracing new beginnings, seizing opportunities, and embracing the beauty of life's ever-changing journey.

Their embrace of new beginnings was a celebration—a celebration of growth, of resilience, and of the infinite potential that love unlocked in their hearts.

XXXV

A Symphony of Love

As Carlos and Isabela embraced new beginnings, they found themselves enveloped in a symphony of love—a harmonious blend of passion, devotion, and the deep connection that defined their relationship.

Their days were filled with moments of intimacy and closeness, as they cherished each other's presence and celebrated the love that bound them together. Carlos's music took on a passionate melody, a reflection of the intensity of their feelings for each other.

One starry night, as they sat on their balcony overlooking the city lights, Carlos and Isabela shared a quiet moment of togetherness. They gazed at the stars above, their hearts overflowing with love and gratitude for the journey they had shared.

Their conversation turned to moments of reflection as they talked about the depth of their love, the ways in which they had grown together, and the dreams they still held dear. Isabela spoke of her admiration for Carlos's unwavering love and support, for being her anchor in times of need and her source of joy in moments of happiness. Carlos, too, expressed his deep affection for Isabela, for the way she had transformed his life with her presence, her love, and her unwavering belief in their future together.

Their words were a symphony—a symphony of love that echoed through the night, a melody that spoke of their commitment, their passion, and the unbreakable bond they shared.

As they held each other close, the city below them bustling with life, Carlos and Isabela felt a sense of completeness. Their love story was not just about overcoming challenges but about the profound connection they had forged, the depth of their emotions, and the beauty of sharing a life filled with love and devotion.

Their symphony of love was a testament—a testament to the enduring power of love, the beauty of true partnership, and the magic of finding your soulmate in a world full of possibilities.

XXXVI

Eternity in a Moment

As Carlos and Isabela basked in the symphony of love, they discovered the timeless beauty of eternity in a moment—a fleeting yet profound glimpse into the depth of their connection and the eternity of their love.

Their days were adorned with moments of pure bliss and contentment, as they savored each moment together and embraced the magic of their bond. Carlos's music took on a transcendent melody, a reflection of the divine harmony they experienced in each other's presence.

One evening, as they sat by the beach, watching the sun dip below the horizon, Carlos and Isabela shared a moment of quiet reverence. They held hands, feeling the warmth of their love enveloping them like a gentle embrace.

Their conversation turned to moments of transcendence as they spoke of the eternal nature of their love, the way it transcended time and space, and the profound connection that defied all boundaries. Isabela spoke of her belief in soulmates, in the idea that their love was destined across lifetimes, and that every moment spent together was a glimpse into eternity. Carlos, too, expressed his conviction that their love was timeless, that it would endure through every challenge and triumph, and that it was a gift beyond measure.

Their words were a prayer—a prayer for eternal love, for moments that stretched into infinity, and for the profound gratitude they felt for finding each other in this vast universe.

As they watched the stars emerge in the night sky, a blanket of twinkling lights above them, Carlos and Isabela felt a sense of awe and wonder. Their love story was not just about the present but about the eternity of their connection, the timeless beauty of their bond, and the knowledge that they were soulmates destined to walk through life together, hand in hand.

Their eternity in a moment was a revelation—a revelation of the boundless nature of love, the sacredness of true partnership, and the endless possibilities that awaited them in the journey ahead.

XXXVII

A Promise of Forever

As Carlos and Isabela embraced the eternity in a moment, they made a promise of forever—a commitment to love each other unconditionally, to cherish every moment, and to build a future filled with happiness and love.

Their days were filled with a sense of purpose and determination, as they looked ahead to the endless possibilities that awaited them. Carlos's music took on a hopeful and resolute melody, a reflection of their steadfast dedication to each other.

One sunny morning, as they walked hand in hand through a garden blooming with flowers, Carlos and Isabela shared their dreams for the future. They spoke of building a home together, of creating a family filled with love and laughter, and of facing life's challenges with courage and resilience.

Their conversation turned to moments of commitment as they expressed their vows to each other, promising to be there in sickness and in health, in joy and in sorrow, and to always support and uplift each other. Isabela spoke of her deep love for Carlos, of her gratitude for the life they were building together, and of her excitement for the journey ahead. Carlos, too, poured his heart out, promising to always cherish and protect Isabela, to be her rock and her partner in every adventure.

Their words were a pledge—a pledge of love, of devotion, and of the unbreakable bond they shared.

As they stood under a canopy of trees, the sunlight filtering through the leaves, Carlos and Isabela felt a sense of peace and fulfillment. Their love story was not just about the present but about the promise of a future filled with love, laughter, and endless possibilities.

Their promise of forever was a testament—a testament to the depth of their love, the strength of their commitment, and the beauty of a love story that would last a lifetime and beyond.

XXXVIII
Embracing the Journey Ahead

As Carlos and Isabela made a promise of forever, they embraced the journey ahead with excitement, anticipation, and a deep sense of gratitude for the love they shared.

Their days were filled with preparations for the future, as they planned their wedding and envisioned the life they would build together. Carlos's music took on a celebratory melody, a reflection of the joy and happiness that filled their hearts.

One evening, as they sat together in their cozy living room, surrounded by photographs of their journey, Carlos and Isabela reminisced about the moments that had brought them to this point. They laughed at the funny mishaps and cherished the sweet memories, feeling grateful for every twist and turn that had led them to each other.

Their conversation turned to moments of gratitude as they expressed their appreciation for the love and support they had received from family and friends. Isabela spoke of the joy of having Carlos by her side, of the laughter they shared, and of the strength they found in each other during difficult times. Carlos, too, shared his gratitude for Isabela, for her unwavering love and for being his partner in every sense of the word.

Their words were a celebration—a celebration of love, of unity, and of the bond that would carry them through all the adventures life had in store.

As they looked at each other, their eyes filled with love and determination, Carlos and Isabela felt a deep sense of peace and happiness. Their love story was not just about the past but about the journey they were embarking upon together, hand in hand, ready to face whatever came their way.

Their embrace of the journey ahead was a promise—a promise to cherish each moment, to support each other through thick and thin, and to build a life filled with love, laughter, and endless possibilities.

XXXIX

A New Chapter Begins

As Carlos and Isabela embraced the journey ahead, they felt a sense of anticipation and excitement for the new chapter unfolding in their lives—a chapter filled with love, laughter, and endless possibilities.

Their days were a whirlwind of activity as they prepared for their wedding, surrounded by family and friends who shared in their joy. Carlos's music filled the air with a festive melody, a reflection of the happiness and celebration that permeated their days.

One bright afternoon, as they finalized the last details for their special day, Carlos and Isabela took a moment to pause and reflect. They stood together in the garden, the sun casting a golden glow around them, and shared a quiet moment of gratitude for everything that had led them to this moment.

Their conversation turned to moments of reflection as they spoke of their journey together, the challenges they had overcome, and the love that had grown stronger with each passing day. Isabela expressed her excitement for the wedding, for the chance to officially start their life together as husband and wife, surrounded by loved ones. Carlos, too, shared his joy and anticipation, grateful for the love and happiness Isabela had brought into his life.

Their words were a vow—a vow of love, of commitment, and of the promise to cherish each other for eternity.

As they stood under the blooming flowers, the scent of fresh blooms filling the air, Carlos and Isabela felt a sense of peace and fulfillment. Their love story was not just about their journey so far but about the endless possibilities that lay ahead, the dreams they would fulfill together, and the life they would build as partners in love and in life.

Their new chapter was a celebration—a celebration of love, of unity, and of the beautiful journey that awaited them as they stepped into the future hand in hand, ready to write the next chapter of their love story.

XL

Love's Eternal Dance

As Carlos and Isabela stood on the brink of a new chapter in their lives, they felt the rhythm of love's eternal dance—a dance that intertwined their hearts, souls, and dreams in a beautiful symphony of togetherness.

Their days leading up to the wedding were filled with excitement and anticipation, as they surrounded themselves with the love and support of their families and friends. Carlos's music echoed the joyous melodies of celebration, a testament to the happiness that enveloped them.

On the eve of their wedding day, as they took a quiet stroll along the beach, Carlos and Isabela reflected on the journey that had brought them to this moment. They shared stories of laughter, tears, and growth, reminiscing about the milestones they had crossed together.

Their conversation turned to moments of gratitude as they expressed their appreciation for the love they had found in each other. Isabela spoke of the way Carlos had brought light into her life, of his unwavering support and understanding. Carlos, too, poured his heart out, thanking Isabela for her love, her kindness, and the way she had made every day feel like a gift.

Their words were a dance—a dance of love that twirled and swayed, carrying them closer together with each step.

As they stood by the water's edge, the moon casting a gentle glow upon them, Carlos and Isabela felt a deep sense of peace and fulfillment. Their love story was not just about the wedding day but about the lifelong journey they had embarked upon, the promise of forever in each other's arms.

Their eternal dance of love was a celebration—a celebration of the bond they shared, the dreams they had woven together, and the endless joy of being united in love, now and for always.

XLI

A Celebration of Love

As Carlos and Isabela stood on the threshold of their wedding day, they were surrounded by a palpable sense of joy and excitement—a celebration of love that echoed through the hearts of everyone who knew them.

The final preparations for the wedding were a flurry of activity, with friends and family coming together to ensure every detail was perfect. Carlos's music filled the air with melodies of happiness and anticipation, setting the stage for a day they would cherish forever.

On the morning of their wedding, as they got ready in separate rooms, Carlos and Isabela exchanged heartfelt letters expressing their love and gratitude. They reminisced about their journey together, from the moment they met to the challenges they had overcome, and the love that had blossomed between them.

Their conversation turned to moments of reflection as they prepared to say "I do." Isabela spoke of her excitement to become Carlos's wife, to walk beside him in all of life's adventures, and to share in the joy of building a future together. Carlos, too, shared his anticipation, grateful for the love and happiness Isabela had brought into his life, and eager to take this next step in their journey.

Their words were a testament—a testament to the love they shared, the promises they made to each other, and the commitment to stand by each other's side through thick and thin.

As they stood at the altar, surrounded by loved ones and the beauty of nature, Carlos and Isabela felt a deep sense of unity and bliss. Their love story was not just about the wedding day but about the journey they had taken together, the growth they had experienced, and the strength of their bond that had only grown stronger with time.

Their celebration of love was a testament—a testament to the power of love, the beauty of commitment, and the joy of finding your soulmate in a world full of possibilities.

XLII

Forever Begins Today

As Carlos and Isabela exchanged vows and sealed their love with a kiss, they embarked on a journey where every moment felt like a new beginning—a testament to the endless possibilities of love and the beauty of shared dreams.

Their wedding day was a celebration of love and unity, with friends and family coming together to witness their commitment. Carlos's music filled the air with melodies of happiness and hope, reflecting the joy that radiated from the newlywed couple.

After the wedding festivities, as they sat together under the starry sky, Carlos and Isabela reflected on the significance of the day. They spoke of their promises to each other, of the dreams they shared, and of the life they envisioned building together.

Their conversation turned to moments of anticipation as they looked forward to their future adventures. Isabela spoke of her excitement for their honeymoon in a secluded beach paradise, where they could bask in each other's love without any distractions. Carlos, too, shared his eagerness to explore new destinations with Isabela, to create memories that would last a lifetime.

Their words were a commitment—a commitment to nurture their love, to face challenges together, and to always prioritize their bond above all else.

As they gazed into each other's eyes, the warmth of their love enveloping them, Carlos and Isabela felt a deep sense of contentment.

Their love story was not just about the wedding day but about the journey that lay ahead, filled with adventures, laughter, and the unwavering support they offered each other.

Their forever began today—a promise of love, a journey of growth, and a lifetime of happiness in each other's arms.

XLIII

Whispers of Tomorrow

As Carlos and Isabela embarked on their honeymoon in the secluded beach paradise, they were enveloped in a world of tranquility and love, where every whisper of the ocean seemed to echo the promises of tomorrow.

Their days were filled with blissful moments of togetherness, as they explored the pristine beaches hand in hand and savored the beauty of nature around them. Carlos's music accompanied their adventures, a melodic backdrop to the harmony of their love.

One evening, as they watched the sun set over the horizon, painting the sky in hues of orange and pink, Carlos and Isabela sat in quiet reflection. They spoke of their dreams for the future, of the family they hoped to build, and of the adventures they wanted to experience together.

Their conversation turned to moments of vision as they discussed their goals and aspirations. Isabela shared her desire to travel the world with Carlos, to discover new cultures and create memories that would last a lifetime. Carlos, too, expressed his dreams of building a home filled with love and laughter, a sanctuary where they could always find peace and happiness.

Their words were a vision—a vision of a future filled with love, laughter, and endless possibilities.

As they walked along the shore, the gentle breeze whispering through their hair, Carlos and Isabela felt a sense of serenity and excitement. Their love story was not just about the honeymoon but about the lifelong journey they were embarking upon, hand in hand, ready to face whatever the future held with courage and love.

Their whispers of tomorrow were a promise—a promise to cherish each moment, to support each other's dreams, and to always believe in the magic of their love story.

XLIV

Capturing Moments

As Carlos and Isabela continued their honeymoon in the secluded beach paradise, they found themselves immersed in a world of beauty and tranquility, capturing each moment as if it were a precious gem in the tapestry of their love story.

Their days were spent exploring the hidden gems of the island, from secret coves with crystal-clear waters to lush rainforests teeming with life. Carlos's music provided a melodic soundtrack to their adventures, a reminder of the harmony they found in each other's company.

One afternoon, as they hiked to a breathtaking viewpoint overlooking the ocean, Carlos and Isabela paused to take in the awe-inspiring scenery. They marveled at the vastness of the sea, the colors of the sky, and the feeling of being connected to something greater than themselves.

Their conversation turned to moments of wonder as they reflected on the beauty of the world around them. Isabela spoke of her appreciation for the simple joys in life, like the warmth of the sun on her skin and the sound of waves crashing against the shore. Carlos, too, shared his awe for nature's wonders, feeling grateful to experience it all with Isabela by his side.

Their words were a testament—a testament to the magic of being present in the moment, to finding joy in the little things, and to the deep bond they shared.

As they sat together, watching the sun dip below the horizon, Carlos and Isabela felt a profound sense of gratitude and love. Their love story was not just about grand gestures but about the quiet moments of connection, the shared experiences that strengthened their bond, and the memories they would carry with them forever.

Their journey of capturing moments was a celebration—a celebration of life, love, and the extraordinary beauty of being together in this world.

XLV

Embracing Serendipity

As Carlos and Isabela continued their honeymoon adventure, they found themselves embracing serendipity in unexpected ways, discovering new joys and surprises that added depth to their journey together.

Their days on the island were filled with exploration and spontaneity, as they wandered through colorful markets, sampled local delicacies, and stumbled upon hidden gems off the beaten path. Carlos's music infused each moment with a sense of wonder and excitement, mirroring the magic they found in each other's presence.

One evening, as they dined at a seaside restaurant, Carlos and Isabela found themselves in the midst of a spontaneous dance under the stars. With the music playing softly in the background, they twirled and laughed, caught up in the joy of the moment and the enchantment of being together.

Their conversation turned to moments of serendipity as they reflected on the unexpected joys life had brought their way. Isabela spoke of the way their love had unfolded organically, like a beautiful dance, each step leading them closer to each other. Carlos, too, shared his appreciation for the twists and turns that had brought them to this magical place, grateful for every serendipitous moment that had shaped their love story.

Their words were a celebration—a celebration of the unexpected, the spontaneous, and the joy of embracing life's surprises.

As they watched the moon cast a shimmering reflection on the ocean, Carlos and Isabela felt a deep sense of connection and gratitude. Their love story was not just about planned adventures but about the magic of spontaneity, the beauty of being in sync with each other, and the joy of discovering new aspects of their love with every passing day.

Their embrace of serendipity was a testament—a testament to the beauty of being open to life's surprises, to the magic of shared moments, and to the endless possibilities of their love story.

XLVI

Echoes of Laughter II

As Carlos and Isabela's honeymoon unfolded, they found themselves surrounded by echoes of laughter, moments of pure joy that filled their days with warmth and happiness, deepening the bond between them.

Their time on the island was a blend of exploration and relaxation, with lazy days spent lounging on the beach, enjoying leisurely walks, and immersing themselves in the vibrant culture of the region. Carlos's music added a playful rhythm to their adventures, a reflection of the laughter that echoed between them.

One afternoon, as they joined a local festival celebrating music and dance, Carlos and Isabela found themselves caught up in the infectious energy of the crowd. They danced with abandon, laughing freely, and reveling in the joy of being alive and together in that moment.

Their conversation turned to moments of laughter as they shared funny anecdotes and silly jokes, their laughter mingling with the sounds of the festivities around them. Isabela spoke of the way Carlos's humor brightened her days, his playful spirit adding a spark of joy to even the simplest moments. Carlos, too, expressed his gratitude for Isabela's laughter, finding solace and happiness in the sound of her joy.

Their words were a melody—a melody of laughter and love, a symphony of happiness that echoed through their hearts.

As they watched the sun set on another perfect day, Carlos and Isabela felt a deep sense of contentment and connection. Their love story was not just about romantic gestures but about the everyday moments of laughter, the shared jokes, and the joy of being able to be themselves completely with each other.

Their echoes of laughter were a celebration—a celebration of love, laughter, and the beautiful music they created together, a melody that would continue to play throughout their lives.

XLVII

Whispers of Tomorrow

As Carlos and Isabela's honeymoon continued, they found themselves immersed in whispers of tomorrow, a gentle reminder of the dreams they shared and the promises they held dear, deepening their connection with each passing day.

Their days on the island were a blend of adventure and tranquility, with mornings spent exploring hidden beaches and afternoons lost in quiet moments of reflection. Carlos's music provided a soothing backdrop to their journey, a melody that echoed the serenity of their love.

One evening, as they sat together watching the stars, Carlos and Isabela spoke of their hopes and aspirations for the future. They shared their dreams of building a life together, of creating a home filled with love and laughter, and of growing old side by side, cherishing every moment along the way.

Their conversation turned to moments of vision as they discussed their plans for the years ahead. Isabela spoke of her desire to start a family, to raise children surrounded by love and warmth. Carlos, too, expressed his dreams of success in his music career, of sharing his passion with the world and making a difference through his art.

Their words were a promise—a promise to support each other's dreams, to navigate life's challenges together, and to always find strength in their love.

As they gazed into each other's eyes, the night sky sparkling above them, Carlos and Isabela felt a deep sense of unity and purpose. Their love story was not just about the present but about the endless possibilities of tomorrow, the dreams they would chase together, and the adventures that awaited them on the horizon.

Their whispers of tomorrow were a melody—a melody of hope, love, and the unwavering belief that their journey was just beginning, with countless chapters yet to unfold.

XLVIII

Embracing the Unknown

As Carlos and Isabela's honeymoon came to a close, they found themselves standing at the threshold of new beginnings, ready to embrace the unknown with courage and love, their hearts filled with anticipation for the journey ahead.

Their final days on the island were a mix of nostalgia and excitement, with moments spent revisiting favorite spots and making new memories together. Carlos's music provided a soundtrack to their reflections, a melody that echoed the emotions swirling in their hearts.

One morning, as they watched the sunrise painting the sky in hues of gold and pink, Carlos and Isabela spoke of the adventures that awaited them beyond the horizon. They talked about their plans to travel the world, to explore new cultures and landscapes, and to continue writing the chapters of their love story in different corners of the globe.

Their conversation turned to moments of anticipation as they shared their eagerness for what the future held. Isabela spoke of the joy of discovering new places with Carlos by her side, of experiencing the wonders of the world together. Carlos, too, expressed his excitement for the journey ahead, knowing that every step they took together would be an adventure worth living.

Their words were a promise—a promise to embrace the unknown, to face challenges with resilience, and to never lose sight of the love that bound them together.

As they packed their bags, ready to leave the island and embark on the next chapter of their lives, Carlos and Isabela felt a sense of exhilaration and gratitude. Their love story was not just about the past or the present but about the endless possibilities that lay ahead, waiting to be discovered, experienced, and cherished.

Their embrace of the unknown was a celebration—a celebration of love, growth, and the excitement of a future filled with infinite possibilities.

XLIX

A New Horizon

As Carlos and Isabela embarked on their journey beyond the island, they were filled with a sense of anticipation and excitement, eager to explore new horizons and write the next chapter of their love story together.

Their first stop on their travels was a bustling city known for its vibrant culture and lively atmosphere. Carlos's music continued to be the soundtrack of their adventures, a reminder of the harmony they found in each other's company.

One day, as they wandered through colorful markets and sampled local delicacies, Carlos and Isabela found themselves caught up in the energy of the city. They marveled at the sights and sounds around them, feeling a sense of wonder and awe at the diversity of the world they were discovering together.

Their conversation turned to moments of exploration as they discussed their plans for the coming months. Isabela spoke of her excitement for the places they would visit, the people they would meet, and the experiences they would share. Carlos, too, expressed his eagerness to immerse himself in new cultures, to learn and grow alongside Isabela as they navigated the adventures of life.

Their words were a journey—a journey of discovery, of growth, and of the endless possibilities that lay before them.

As they watched the sunset over the city skyline, Carlos and Isabela felt a deep sense of gratitude and joy. Their love story was not just about the past or the present but about the ever-evolving journey they were on, together, hand in hand, ready to embrace each new day with open hearts and minds.

Their embrace of the new horizon was a celebration—a celebration of love, adventure, and the beauty of experiencing life's wonders together.

L

Everlasting Love

As Carlos and Isabela continued their journey of exploration and discovery, they found themselves reflecting on the depth and endurance of their love, a love that had grown stronger with each passing day and had weathered every challenge they faced together.

Their travels took them to picturesque landscapes and charming towns, each place leaving a mark on their hearts and deepening their bond. Carlos's music continued to be a constant source of comfort and inspiration, a reminder of the melody of their love story.

One evening, as they sat by a tranquil lake, watching the stars reflected in the water, Carlos and Isabela spoke of their journey—the highs and lows, the laughter and tears, the moments of pure joy and the times of quiet understanding. They marveled at how far they had come, how much they had grown individually and as a couple, and how their love had stood the test of time.

Their conversation turned to moments of reflection as they shared their dreams for the future. Isabela spoke of her hopes for a life filled with love, laughter, and continued adventures with Carlos by her side. Carlos, too, expressed his gratitude for Isabela's unwavering support, her love giving him the strength to pursue his passions and dreams.

Their words were a testament—a testament to the power of love, the beauty of partnership, and the resilience of the human spirit.

As they held hands under the starlit sky, Carlos and Isabela felt a profound sense of peace and contentment. Their love story was not just a collection of moments but a tapestry woven with threads of laughter, tears, dreams, and shared experiences—a tapestry that would continue to unfold and grow richer with each passing year.

Their everlasting love was a celebration—a celebration of the journey they had been on, the love they shared, and the promise of a future filled with endless possibilities, together, forever.

LI

Dreams Unfolding

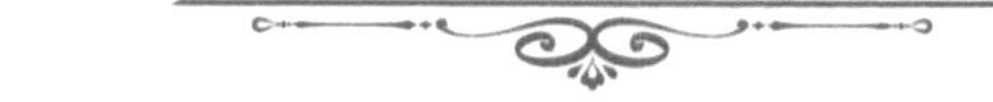

As Carlos and Isabela embraced the beauty of their everlasting love, they found themselves dreaming of new beginnings and exciting adventures yet to come. Their journey together was like a canvas waiting to be painted with the colors of their shared dreams and aspirations.

Their travels led them to a quaint seaside town, where the salty breeze carried whispers of endless possibilities. Carlos's music, infused with the melody of their love story, filled the air as they explored charming cobblestone streets and stumbled upon hidden gems around every corner.

One afternoon, as they sat on a cliff overlooking the ocean, Carlos and Isabela let their imaginations run wild. They talked about their dreams for the future—a cozy home by the sea, filled with laughter and warmth, where they could raise a family and create lifelong memories.

Their conversation turned to moments of anticipation as they envisioned their dreams unfolding. Isabela spoke of the joy of building a life together, of watching their love grow with each passing day. Carlos, too, expressed his excitement for the adventures they would embark on, knowing that their love was the anchor that would guide them through any storm.

Their words were like poetry—a reflection of the beauty they saw in each other and the dreams they shared.

As they watched the sunset paint the sky in hues of pink and orange, Carlos and Isabela felt a sense of wonder and gratitude. Their love story was not just a chapter but a book filled with endless possibilities, a story of two hearts beating as one, ready to embrace whatever the future held.

Their dreams unfolding were a celebration—a celebration of love, hope, and the magic of creating a life together, one dream at a time.

LII

Paths Intertwined

As Carlos and Isabela's journey continued, they found themselves on a path where their destinies intertwined in unexpected ways, revealing the beauty of serendipity and the power of their connection.

Their travels took them to a lively city filled with bustling streets and colorful markets, each corner brimming with stories waiting to be discovered. Carlos's music, a reflection of their shared experiences and emotions, echoed through the vibrant city as they explored its hidden treasures.

One day, as they strolled hand in hand through a charming neighborhood, Carlos and Isabela encountered an old bookstore tucked away in a quiet alley. Intrigued, they stepped inside, greeted by shelves lined with books of all genres and eras.

Their curiosity led them to a section on travel and adventure, where they stumbled upon a worn-out journal filled with handwritten notes and sketches. As they flipped through its pages, they discovered that the journal belonged to a couple who had traveled the world together, capturing moments of love, laughter, and discovery along the way.

Carlos and Isabela were captivated by the stories within the journal, each page a testament to the beauty of shared experiences and the magic of exploring the world as a couple. They felt a connection to the unknown authors, as if their paths had crossed in the pages of the journal, weaving their own story into the tapestry of adventures.

Their conversation turned to moments of reflection as they pondered the paths that had led them to this bookstore, to this moment of discovery. Isabela spoke of the synchronicities that seemed to guide their journey, of the way their lives had intertwined in ways they never could have imagined. Carlos, too, expressed his gratitude for the serendipitous moments that had brought them closer together, knowing that every twist and turn had led them to this beautiful chapter of their lives.

Their words were a symphony—a melody of gratitude, wonder, and the profound realization that their paths were meant to cross, destined to intertwine in a dance of love and adventure.

As they left the bookstore, the sun setting on the horizon, Carlos and Isabela felt a sense of awe and wonder at the mysteries of fate. Their love story was not just a series of moments but a journey of discovery, where every encounter, every discovery, was a reminder of the magic of being together.

Their paths intertwining were a celebration—a celebration of destiny, connection, and the joy of sharing life's adventures with the one you love.

LIII

A Glimpse of Eternity

As Carlos and Isabela continued their journey, they found themselves in a serene coastal town, where the rhythm of the ocean and the whisper of the wind seemed to echo the timeless beauty of their love.

Their days were spent exploring sandy beaches and hidden coves, each moment a precious treasure in the tapestry of their shared experiences. Carlos's music, now intertwined with the sounds of nature, created a symphony that mirrored the depth of their connection.

One evening, as they sat beneath a canopy of stars, Carlos and Isabela gazed out at the vast expanse of the sea. The moon cast a gentle glow on the water, turning it into a shimmering canvas of silver and blue.

Their conversation drifted to moments of eternity as they reflected on the immensity of the universe and the fleeting nature of time. Isabela spoke of the timeless quality of their love, of how every moment spent together felt like a glimpse of eternity. Carlos, too, expressed his awe at the beauty of the night sky, knowing that their love was as infinite as the stars above.

Their words were a meditation—a reflection on the eternal nature of love, the interconnectedness of all things, and the profound sense of peace that comes from being in harmony with the universe.

As they sat in silence, the waves lapping gently at the shore, Carlos and Isabela felt a deep sense of unity with the world around them. Their love story was not just about their bond but about their connection to something greater, something timeless and eternal.

Their glimpse of eternity was a celebration—a celebration of love that transcends time and space, a love that continues to grow and evolve with each passing moment.

LIV

The Invitation

E pilogue:
As Carlos and Isabela's journey came to a close, their hearts were filled with gratitude for the adventures they had shared, the love they had discovered, and the growth they had experienced together. Their love story, like a tapestry woven with threads of laughter, tears, dreams, and shared experiences, had become a testament to the power of love to transform lives.

As they stood on the shore, watching the sun dip below the horizon, Carlos turned to Isabela with a smile. "Our story doesn't end here," he said, his eyes sparkling with excitement. "It's just the beginning of a new chapter."

Isabela nodded, her heart filled with anticipation for the future. "Every sunset is a promise of a new dawn," she replied, taking Carlos's hand in hers.

And so, dear readers, I invite you to join Carlos and Isabela on the next chapter of their journey—a journey filled with new adventures, dreams yet to be realized, and the endless possibilities that love brings. As their story continues to unfold, may you find inspiration in their love, courage in their resilience, and joy in their shared moments.

For love is not just a destination but a journey—a journey of discovery, growth, and the beauty of being truly seen and loved.

Thank you for being a part of "Unexpected Romance in Rio." May your own love story be filled with wonder, passion, and the magic of endless possibilities.

The End.

Closing Curtain: Love's Rhythm In Rio

Dear Reader,

As we come to the end of "Unexpected Romance in Rio," I am filled with gratitude for the opportunity to share Carlos and Isabela's journey with you. This story has been a labor of love, and I hope it has touched your heart and kindled your imagination.

To me, storytelling is a way of weaving together the threads of our shared human experiences, of celebrating love in all its forms, and of finding beauty in the unexpected moments that shape our lives.

I want to express my deepest thanks to everyone who has been a part of this book's creation—from the characters who came to life on these pages to the readers who embarked on this adventure with an open heart.

May "Unexpected Romance in Rio" remind you that love is a force that transcends barriers, a source of strength in times of uncertainty, and a beacon of hope that guides us through life's twists and turns.

With heartfelt gratitude,

Mikey Katodiya

Also by Mikey

Love Stories Around the World
First Love in Paris
Lost Love in Tokyo
Unexpected Romance in Rio

Watch for more at oximefx@gmail.com.

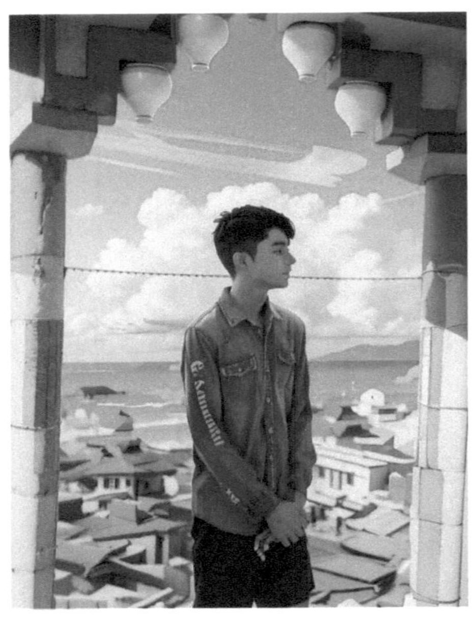

About the Author

Meet, who often goes by the pen name "Mikey," is a passionate writer who believes in the power of storytelling to inspire and heal. Writing has been his creative outlet, allowing him to explore complex emotions and share them with others. 'Yesterday's Love Story' is his debut work, born frompersonal experiences and a desire to connect with readers on a deeply emotional level. Meet hopes his words, written under the pen nameMikey, will resonate with those seeking solace and strength in the face of adversity.

Read more at https://www.instagram.com/bigpicstory.